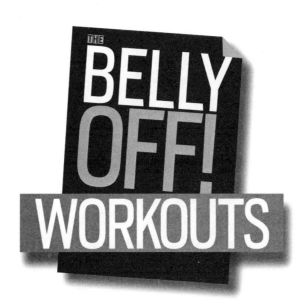

THE
BELLY
OFF!
WORKOUTS

# THE BELLY OFF! WORKOUTS

## A 6-WEEK DETOX DIET AND FITNESS PLAN THAT STRIPS AWAY FAT—FAST!

**JEFF CSATARI** and **DAVID JACK** WITH THE EDITORS OF **Men'sHealth**

© 2013 by Rodale Inc.
Trade paperback and exclusive direct online hardcover published simultaneously by Rodale Inc.

Rodale books may be purchased for business or promotional use or for special sales.
For information, please write to:
Special Markets Department, Rodale Inc., 733 Third Avenue, New York, NY 10017.

*Men's Health* is a registered trademark of Rodale Inc.
Printed in the United States of America

Rodale Inc. makes every effort to use acid-free ♾, recycled paper ♻.

Photographs by Tom MacDonald


Library of Congress Cataloging-in-Publication Data is on file with the publisher.

ISBN-13: 978–1–60961–876–6 paperback


Distributed to the trade by Macmillan

2   4   6   8   10   9   7   5   3   1   paperback

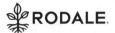

We inspire and enable people to improve their lives and the world around them

**rodalebooks.com**

TO THE BELLY OFF! CLUB MEMBERS

# CONTENTS

PART 3
# BELLY OFF! NUTRITION

PART 4
# THE FAT BURNER'S BAG OF TRICKS

# ACKNOWLEDGMENTS

**W**e at *Men's Health* firmly believe that it's never too late to get back in shape. With the right plan and a little gumption, you can change your body and improve your health—dramatically. This book will help you to succeed not only because it's a proven program but also because it was created by a team of smart and talented people—folks who've got your back. I thank them all and recognize some of them here.

David Jack for his infectious enthusiasm for fitness and skill in developing great workouts, and Belly Off! nutrition expert Chris Mohr, RD, PhD, of MohrResults.com, for his diet and weight-loss wisdom.

The entire editorial team at Rodale books; in particular, Stephen Perrine, Beth Lamb, George Karabotsos, Chris Rhoads, Debbie McHugh, Chris Krogermeier, Sara Cox, Nancy Bailey, Liz Krenos, and Thomas MacDonald.

David Zinczenko and those always-helpful friends at *Men's Health* magazine, and Belly Off! trainer Craig Ballantyne.

My best friend, Kathy, and our daughters, Katelyn, Lydia, and Sophia. And to my Csatari cousins for loaning me that homemade wooden bench and those cement barbells when I was 10.

—Jeff Csatari

**I** believe it's becoming rare in life to find a career that you enjoy, can use to help others, and in turn experience great fulfillment. I have been blessed to find a path that allows me to do just that.

So many people have shaped me personally and professionally. I am sincerely grateful to them and would like to offer special thanks to:

My mom, Donna, and dad, Duff (RIP), for providing me the structure and the freedom to pursue my dreams; to my wife, Wendy, for her unconditional support and love (I am so proud of you); her mom and dad, Sharon and Rene, for theirs; and to my beautiful daughters, Ava and Ella, who make me better and fill me with love everyday.

BJ Baker and Mike Morris for their mentorship; Tony and Daral for their sage wisdom and their lifesaving invitations; to my peers who have challenged me and made me a better coach, especially my original team at Teamworks/CATZ: Jeremy, Donnell, Shane, Mike, and Tammy.

My brother Donny, Dave G, Jeremy S, Brian W, Mickey P, JD, Luke, Chad, Dan, and Josh—what a blessing it is to "walk" with you.

The editors of *Men's Health* and *Women's Health* magazines, especially Adam Campbell, Jeff Csatari, Kevin Donahue, and Bill Stump. Also to the Belly Off! community—your courage, stories, and inspiration have truly been a gift in my life.

A special professional thanks goes out to Reebok, Perform Better, and the International Youth Conditioning Association for their trust in me and for adding value to my life.

Finally to the Lord for His provision and grace in my life, for making human beings the greatest miracles in the world, and for choosing and equipping me to work with them.

—David Jack

# INTRODUCTION

A lot of guys want six-pack abs. A lot of guys also want baby back ribs. (Extra barbecue sauce, please.) The problem is, one kind of six-pack never leads to the other. You know what I mean. It's not so easy to have the abs if you make a habit of beer and ribs. That's reality, friend. Need a napkin?

When you see a shirtless actor on the big screen sporting washboard abs, you can bet he hasn't been sucking down longnecks, pork barbecue, and hush puppies. How about the actress in the skimpy two-piece bouncing in the surf for the paparazzi? She probably spent the morning strapped into a Pilates reformer. Check out her . . . *obliques!*

Despite what many of the diet books may promise, losing weight takes a bit of effort and acceptance of those scary concepts known as *discipline* and *sacrifice*. If there's a magic bullet to shedding belly fat—and there really isn't any magic to it—it's accepting the fact that you have to make some changes in your life if you're going to change your body. A turnaround results from doing something different. Success starts by identifying what that change needs to be.

The Belly Off! Club is filled with hundreds of thousands of people who did just that over the past 12 years. Driven by a "wake-up call" in their lives or inspired by others' success, they all did the same thing—they put their finger on exactly what was holding them back from living the life they really wanted. And then they set out to do something about it.

The change didn't come overnight, and they will be the first to tell you that. It happened gradually, in baby steps, and often with setbacks—those doses of reality that anyone embarking on a challenge should expect. But it always happened with conviction.

"I knew I had to get back in shape," recalls Jeff Atwater, a Belly Off! Club member from Massachusetts. "But it wasn't until I recognized

**"Exercise is now a part of who I am."**

—Jeff Atwater,
The Belly Off! Club, 2010

how good I felt about myself after losing weight and how amazing my physical self felt after every workout that I became convinced that this was the new me. Exercise is now a part of who I am."

If you've read *The Belly Off! Diet* or joined our online club, you may know the story of Belly Off! For those who are new to the club, here's a brief time line of how Belly Off! came to be. Like a lot of ideas here at magazine and book publisher Rodale Inc., it grew, well, organically . . .

A bunch of *Men's Health* magazine editors had just finished their regular Wednesday noontime basketball game. Shirts versus skins. And one sweaty editor said, "Ya know, we doughboys don't look anything like the buff dudes on the cover of our magazine."

The lightbulbs came on—instant story idea: We'll hire a trainer and a nutritionist to put us on a 6-week program to turn our bodies around and, we hope, help us find our abs. The story about our journey ran in the October 2000 issue. In it, you'll read that some of us did see our abs emerge, but all of us improved our health and discovered muscles we didn't know we had. In that same article, we invited readers to join the Belly Off! Club at menshealth.com and transform their bodies, too. And they did. In droves. That was more than 12 years ago. Since then, we've featured a Belly Off! success story in almost every issue of the magazine, and you'll find many more online. All told, well over 300,000 people have used these Belly Off! stories as inspiration to lose more than 2 million pounds and, more important, dramatically improve their health.

And they continue to do so. We encourage you to join the Belly Off! Club at menshealth.com/bellyoff along with following the advice in this book. Start a member profile and use the advice, tips, and member forums to spur your own journey toward a leaner, stronger, healthier body.

## ANOTHER WAKE-UP CALL

I dropped 14 pounds in 3 weeks while testing and developing the Belly Off! Diet and fitness program for the first book back in 2009. Since then, I've kept off most of that weight, having learned and followed the most useful (for me) Belly Off! lesson of all: Stop drinking soda and juice. Make your calories count. Those empty liquid ones aren't worth it.

Working for a publisher of healthy living books and magazines comes with some nice lifestyle perks: We have an excellent company gym right down the street from the office, and it's filled with all the latest fitness gear and offers terrific classes. The cafeteria serves up healthy entrées (many of them taken right out of the weight-loss cookbooks we publish), amazing salads and soups, and lots of organic options. On Friday afternoons, organic farmers sell produce, eggs, cheese, free-range beef, and wild salmon in the company dining hall. If I go for a sweaty afternoon run on the wooded trail right outside our building, my colleagues are grateful that there are employee shower facilities available to me afterward. Plus, I have access to the largest health library and medical journal database on the East Coast (it's just one flight up—always take the stairs!), so I can keep up on the latest health and fitness research. I figure I'm healthier than a lot of guys my age, thanks to spending more than 8 hours a day in a place where you're never far from reminders to eat right and exercise.

All of that sounds great, right? Almost *too* perfect, right?

Right.

Last month, I had a blood test, and the results freaked me out. I'm just about one sugar cookie away from a prediabetes diagnosis. In researching an article I was writing about advanced medical tests for *Men's Health*, I filled a vial with my best red for a test called hemoglobin A1C (or HbA1c, for short). Unlike the fasting glucose test most family docs routinely use (a test that is fairly inaccurate, for the record), this test measures your average blood sugar over 3 months, giving you a far better picture of how well your body is processing sugar over an extended period of time. The doctor described it like so: Glucose molecules adhere to your red blood cells like sugar to a doughnut. The more sugar, the worse it gets. I guess I had quite a few of these *hemo-goblins*, because my numbers were pretty scary. Over time, the glucose causes damage to your heart, brain, kidneys, eyes, and nerves.

Prediabetes? My family doctor didn't seem that concerned because my HbA1c score was right on the borderline. But it genuinely scared me. I know that prediabetes is just a step away from full-blown diabetes, and most people with "pre" eventually get to "D." I remember what Florence Comite, MD, an endocrinologist I interviewed some time ago told me about HbA1c: "It's one of the best tests of longevity."

And I just failed it.

Diabetes is a horrifying disease, which often leads those who cannot manage it properly down an icy slope toward heart disease, stroke, blindness, amputation, cancer, and premature death. It is arguably the single biggest health epidemic of our time. Experts estimate that by 2020 it will affect one in two Americans. Here's another stat that may make you reconsider that croissant: Gaining 17 pounds triples your likelihood of developing diabetes. And another: Most prediabetics, upward of 33 million in the United States, like me, don't know they have it.

That's what really blew my mind: I didn't have a clue. Here I am, thinking I'm doing all right for a middle-age guy. I'm exercising at least four times a week. I still fit into my size 34 jeans. If I didn't have this blood test, I wouldn't know I'm on the verge of prediabetes (aka metabolic syndrome). I'd think everything was hunky-dory. Thank goodness I had that blood test. Now I know what I have to deal with—sugar-coated hemoglobin. It's my *new* wake-up call. And I'm going to answer it with a renewed effort to clean up my diet of pasta, rice, bread, and baked goods and tackle the *new* metabolic workouts my friend and colleague David Jack has designed for us—workouts contained right here in this book. Fortunately, prediabetes is pretty simple to make go away. Even full-blown type 2 diabetes can be reversed, sometimes without drugs, through diligent dietary changes, exercise, and weight loss.

Where do you stand? Think you're doing all right? Even if your waistline isn't bulging over your belt, I encourage you to ask your doctor about an HbA1c blood test to check your blood sugar. If your belly is big, make an appointment with your doctor today and demand this test.

Diabetes is a poisonous snake at your feet that you can't see or hear; you don't even know it's there—until it strikes.

Your next step? Turn the page and make a pact with yourself to follow the Belly Off! Code of Conduct, the six simple principles that will have a dramatic impact on your belly size and your overall health. These principles are supported by the meat of this book:

- The new Belly Off! 2-Minute Drill, a morning ritual that will kick your metabolism into high gear.

- The Belly Off! 6-Week Detox, a 12-point nutrition plan that will whisk "the white stuff" from your diet, burn fat, and fuel your body for the workout program.

- The Belly Off! Walking Program with a 14-Day Kick Start, which quickly constructs a foundation of fitness to build upon.

- New Belly Off! Recipes, which will help you make meals to resuscitate your taste buds when you tire of chicken breast.

- The Belly Off! Back-in-Shape Workouts, innovative metabolism-boosting, strength-building exercise routines designed to help you shed dangerous belly fat fast, featuring a special workout custom-made for beginners.

- Advanced workouts, including progressive programs that help you achieve the body you've always wanted.

Finally, this book is chock-full of tips, advice, and inspiration from Belly Off! Club members who've made the lifestyle changes and reaped the healthy rewards that you can earn, too, with the right plan, with the Belly Off! Workouts.

—Jeff Csatari

P.S. It starts with a commitment.

On the next page, you will find the Belly Off! Club Code of Conduct. Read it. Sign it. Date it. Follow it. Making a promise to yourself is the secret serum that will melt your Belly Off!

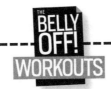

# THE BELLY OFF! CLUB
# CODE OF CONDUCT

## I PROMISE TO ...

■ **Eat breakfast every day.**

It will be rich in protein and include some fats and slow-burning carbohydrates.

■ **Exercise daily.**

Do the Belly Off! 2-Minute Drill every morning, follow the walking program, and perform a Belly Off! strength workout three times per week.

■ **Eliminate sweet beverages.**

That includes fruit juices, sodas, teas with added sugar, and flavored coffee.

■ **Enjoy four to six small meals a day.**

Try to include some protein and fiber each time. Refueling this way will raise your metabolism, keep blood sugar levels stable, and prevent overeating.

■ **Cut out processed carbohydrates.**

Remove cakes, cookies, chips, crackers, white bread, pasta, white rice, ice cream, and candy from your diet. Replace them with fresh vegetables and fruits, legumes, whole grains, nuts, seeds, lean protein, and satiating fats.

■ **Avoid alcohol for 6 weeks.**

No beer, wine, or cocktails. This is the easiest way to cut calories and burn fat fast.

**Signed:** _____ **Date:** _____

# PART
# 1

## THE WARMUP

If you are a beginner, Part 1 The Warmup is custom-made for you. This kickoff to the Back-in-Shape Workouts includes lifestyle, diet, and fitness boosters to get you going, a walking interval program, including an easy, start-from-scratch 14-day walking plan, and an introduction to new Belly Off! 2-Minute Drills of low-impact bodyweight exercises. Simply by moving your body more every day, you will burn calories, increase your flexibility, and lay a foundation for fitness. The program has built-in progressions that push you a little bit more each time you work out. That way, you gradually build strength and cardiovascular endurance. The regimen is ideal for those who are significantly overweight or even obese. We've teamed it with a 6-week detox plan, detailed in Part 3, that will clean up your diet and provide the nutrition needed to support your workouts. Good nutrition fuels your exercise. Regular exercise maximizes good nutrition. Both work together to speed weight loss. If you're not significantly overweight and are simply looking to get back in shape, Part 1 is still a great place for you to start.

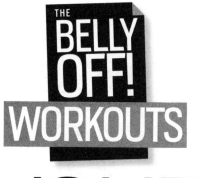

# Chapter 1

# YOUR BELLY OFF! BOOSTERS

## 5 Steps to Start Changing Your Life Today!

Welcome to *The Belly Off! Workouts*, where the fat meets the fire. Inside this book you will find extremely effective exercise routines and nutrition advice that will help you to look, feel, and live better than ever. Begin your journey right here, right now with these life-altering boosters.

The goal of the Belly Off! Workouts is to start chipping away at your midsection. We really do want to take your belly off! It's not just an issue of appearance and comfort—sporting a big belly has real implications for your health. It is a medical fact that the bigger your middle, the higher your risk of disease.

Belly fat is called visceral fat because it collects deep underneath your abdominal muscle layer, around your internal organs. It's fat that doesn't jiggle, but presses out your middle, giving you that apple-shaped body. A waist circumference over 40 inches for men and 35 for women is a major risk factor for type 2 diabetes. In fact, most endocrinologists can guess with 90 percent accuracy whether or not you have prediabetes by simply looking at the size of your belly. That's how easy it is to spot this kind of dangerous fat. Visceral fat interferes with insulin production and blood sugar regulation, and it secretes chemicals that trigger inflammation that contributes to type 2 diabetes.

A large midsection is also implicated in high blood pressure, depression, sexual dysfunction, cancer, and—of course—heart disease. A study at the University of Alabama-Birmingham looked at several different factors that determine a person's heart disease risk. The researchers found that the biggest single predictor of a heart attack in a person's future is the amount of visceral fat in his or her abdomen.

We understand that you may be eager to look great in a bathing suit or new work clothes, and Belly Off! will get you there—but our first priority is to improve your health. Conveniently, shedding your belly using the strategies in this book will help you achieve both goals at the same time.

During the next 6 weeks, even if you're an absolute beginner, you will construct a solid base of fitness and begin to significantly transform the look and shape of your body. You'll have more energy. You'll be happier. Your friends and family will look up to you as someone who has taken charge of his life, someone who is active, healthy, and in control. If you have any doubt that you have what it takes to succeed on this program, remember this: A strong work ethic is the great equalizer. If you work consistently and follow the advice in this book, don't worry—you *will* achieve your goal of reducing your belly size and improving your health. We've made it very easy to start: Just use the boosters discussed below and remember to make a pact with yourself using the Belly Off! Club Code of Conduct (see page xvi). Having a plan and working toward a goal has been the secret sauce for success for hundreds of thousands of Belly Off! Club members, and it will work for you.

Now, before you lace up your running shoes, we want you to grab a pen for the first step in your five-point jump start.

## BOOSTER #1:
## START A FOOD DIARY

On page 15, you'll find a food diary that we recommend you fill out at the start of your get-back-in-shape program. The reason? To help convince you that your diet needs to change at the same time that your activity level does. Exercise alone won't cut it. No Belly Off! Club member lost 15 pounds or more without altering his food intake—the biggest modifiable factor in your effort to gain fitness. We want you to be conscious of what you are putting in your mouth so you'll have a clear picture of what needs to change. There is no better way of doing that than by keeping a food diary for at least 3 days. Make copies of the sample log on page 15. Here are a few helpful tips to keep in mind while filling it in.

**FITNESS**

## What Kind of Exercise Results in the Most Weight Loss?

Here are the top five answers of the Belly Off! Club online:

**1.** The kind you will do every day.

**2.** Any fast-paced workout.

**3.** The exercise that you find most enjoyable to stick with.

**4.** Interval training.

**5.** Circuit-style weight lifting with exercises that work the most muscles.

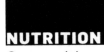

## NUTRITION
## Start with a Shake

Drinking a protein shake before and during a weight-training session may speed weight loss and help build lean muscle, according to researchers at Syracuse University. They found that people who drank a combination of amino acids and carbohydrates had higher metabolic rates the next day compared with when they ate only carbs. People in the test reaped this benefit after drinking a shake containing 22 grams of protein mixed with 35 grams of carbohydrates.

■ **Choose 3 consecutive days to keep track of your food intake, and make sure at least 1 of those days falls on a weekend.** Why? Because Saturday and Sunday are the days when people eat the most food. A study at Washington University School of Medicine found that the average American consumes 236 more calories on a weekend day than on a weekday. That can add up to a 9-pound weight gain over the course of a year. It's beneficial to know how much more you're eating on your days off and how that figure changes depending on how you spend your weekend.

■ **Eat normally.** Don't try to be "good." You want to paint an accurate picture of your regular diet. Jot down what and roughly how much you've eaten after every main meal. At the same time, include any snacks that you've eaten between meals. (Recording your food intake just three times a day instead of after every morsel you consume simply makes the food diary task less of a hassle and easier to keep up with.)

■ **Be sure to track your beverages, too; they're a significant source of empty calories.** Tally the number of glasses of water you drink in a day, as well. You will likely be surprised by how little water you actually consume.

■ **At the end of each day, figure out a rough calorie count for each meal.** (Use a calorie counter book or an online source to quickly guesstimate the calories in each meal.) Tally and record your total daily calories.

After the third day, review your log. How many calories did you consume? From which types of foods did the bulk of your calories come? How much of what you ate was lean protein and fruits and vegetables? How much was processed foods?

How many foods are included in the list of "Foods with the Most Nutrition Per Calorie" versus "Foods with the Least Nutrition Per Calorie" on page 8? We guarantee this little exercise will be an eye-opener and will point out exactly what in your diet needs to change. You may find that it's so helpful that you'll want to continue keeping track of your meals.

## BOOSTER #2:
## START CLEANING UP YOUR DIET

Unless it happens to be a real blueberry, stay away from blue food. Blue #2 is an artificial dye used along or mixed with other dyes to color many, many processed foods. Studies involving mice that were fed rodent-appropriate doses of Blue #2 in their food suggest that the chemical can trigger the growth of tumors in the brain and elsewhere. Where do you find Blue #2? In the most heavily processed foods—cereals, candy, cake frosting, etc. But don't go hunting for it on product labels, just start reducing your consumption of food that comes in a box, bag, or can. Keep it simple. Eat fresh.

The next easiest way to clean up your diet is to cut back on drinking soda, juice, or sugary fruit drinks. Your body can't monitor liquid calories well, so it's very easy to consume ridiculous quantities of sugar water and calories without even recognizing the load you are placing on your system. And don't think that diet soda is your savior. A University of North Carolina at Chapel Hill study found that when people swapped their favorite sugary soft drink for the diet variety, they made up for the sacrifice by eating more desserts and more bread than people who drank water. It seems that artificial sweeteners increase your hunger for sweet things, the researchers say.

**IT WORKS FOR ME**

"To overcome tough phases in a weight-loss program, it helps to develop a mantra. Here's mine: 'In your life up until this point, you have been one person. It is time to show the world who you can be.'"

—Andy Hayes
**Weight Before:**
300 pounds
**Weight After:**
190 pounds
The Belly Off! Club,
April 2011

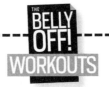

## FOODS WITH THE MOST NUTRITION PER CALORIE

- Eggs
- Almonds
- Avocados
- Spinach
- Salmon
- Turkey
- Cantaloupe
- Mozzarella cheese
- Tomatoes
- Blueberries

## FOODS WITH THE LEAST NUTRITION PER CALORIE

- Sugar
- White rice
- White bread
- Pasta
- Doughnuts
- Potato chips
- Candy
- Soda

The solution? Water. Drink lots of it. If you are a big juice and soda drinker, this change alone will have a significant impact on your weight very quickly.

Another easy way to simplify your diet: Don't add sugar or salt to your foods. You don't need them. Hide the saltshaker and sugar bowl, if you must. Begin cutting back with tomorrow morning's coffee. If you normally use two teaspoons of sugar, use one. If you use one, use a half. Gradually wean yourself off the white stuff. Tip: When making your coffee, sprinkle a pinch of cinnamon into the grounds before you start to brew. You know that caffeine raises your resting metabolic rate. What you may not know is that cinnamon will help to regulate your blood sugar levels, helping to keep fat off your belly.

# BOOSTER #3:
# START EATING MORE
# PROTEIN AND FIBER

In Part 3 of this book, you'll learn just how much protein and fiber you should try to swallow every day for optimum Belly Off! success. But for now, just start making an effort to eat some protein- and fiber-rich food at every meal. Both of these nutrients will fill you up and keep you satisfied longer than carbohydrates will. By eating more, you'll automatically reduce the amount of fast-burning carbs you consume.

Here's a no-brainer way to ensure that you use this Belly Off! booster daily:

Fill half of your breakfast or dinner plate with protein (eggs, beef, chicken, fish, turkey) and half with vegetables or fruit (especially high-fiber varieties). For fruit, focus on raspberries, blackberries, apples, and pears (with skin), which are among the highest in fiber.

If you find it difficult to get enough fiber, consider using a fiber supplement like Metamucil, a psyllium fiber powder that you mix in water or juice. Start with a small amount and increase the dosage gradually. Down a glass before a meal and you'll likely end up feeling full faster.

Another effective dietary supplement to try is PGX granules, made from glucomannan, which has a very high viscosity level. Research has shown that glucomannan can lower your insulin response after a meal by 50 percent, while also lowering bad cholesterol by 20 percent and blood sugar by 23 percent. Mix a scoop into yogurt, juice, or water. In the gut, it expands into a gelatinous mass, making you feel full very quickly. The glucomannan fiber also slows digestion. Taken before a meal, it will lower the glycemic index of any food you eat—so it's a good "appetizer" if you're having pasta. Studies

**NUTRITION**

## Backward Omelets

The protein in whole eggs helps you feel fuller for longer, says Belly Off! nutritionist Christopher Mohr, PhD, RD, of the weight-loss firm Mohr Results. But next time, flip the omelet's vegetable-to-egg ratio: Melt a little butter in a pan over medium-high heat. Add lots of fresh chopped vegetables. Sauté. Add two beaten eggs. Scramble, cook through, and serve.

## Hide Tempting Foods

Having lots of enticing foods in front of your eyes and within reach of your hands will destroy your willpower and derail your weight-loss efforts. You know this. So why is there a bowl of chocolates on your kitchen counter? Or a tin of sugar cookies in your pantry? Have you ever been able to walk past an open bag of potato chips without dipping your hand inside? Remember this about salty and sweet snacks: Out of sight, out of mind, out of belly.

suggest that glucomannan supplementation can cause weight loss even in people who don't restrict calories. In one study, obese adults who took 1 gram of glucomannan fiber an hour before every meal for 8 weeks lost an average of 5.5 pounds without making any other changes to their diet or exercise programs. An earlier study by researchers at the University of Connecticut compared two groups of overweight men and women who were given glucomannan to take 5 minutes before their two largest meals each day. Both groups were put on the same diet, but only one group was asked to do regular exercise. The study found that the exercisers and nonexercisers alike lost the same amount of weight after 8 weeks, suggesting the potential of this fiber to aid weight loss even without exercise. The American Dietetic Association recommends getting 30 grams of fiber a day. Surveys indicate that the average American consumes less than half that amount.

## BOOSTER #4: START ELIMINATING FAST FOOD

This week, eat fewer meals at fast-food restaurants then you did last week. You'll save hundreds of calories simply by eating a few more meals at home. If a daily fast-food run is your habit, cut out two drive-thru visits. If you go three times a week, eliminate one of these stops. Start getting into the habit of preparing breakfast and dinner at home and taking snacks like almonds, apples, cheese sticks, and yogurt to work.

When you do eat at restaurants, take greater control of what you consume. Here are some simple ways to start.

- **When ordering a salad, nix the croutons.** Ask for dressing on the side so you—not a heavy-handed line cook—can determine how much you need.

- **Send back the bread basket.** Or take one piece and send back the rest so you won't be tempted.

- **Order unsweetened iced tea or water with lemon.** You'll eliminate about 200 calories instantly by avoiding soda!

- **Make it an omelet.** If you are going to have a restaurant meal, make it breakfast (or have breakfast for dinner).

# BOOSTER #5:
# START MOVING MORE

You don't *have* to be sweating underneath a barbell to burn calories. When you think about it, the time you spend exercising—even if you do it for a full hour—counts for just a fraction of your activity during your waking day. The real trick to burning more calories is to bump up your natural movement throughout the day.

If you sit for a living—that is, at a desk in front of a computer, like a lot of people do—that can be challenging. But it's not an insurmountable problem. In fact, it doesn't take much effort to make a difference. A recent study in the journal *Medicine and Science in Sports and Exercise* showed that it takes just 30 total daily minutes of "incidental moderate physical activity" (that would be taking the stairs instead of the elevator) to improve long-term health and fitness. Here are some basic move-more habits that we know you've heard before but could probably benefit from hearing again.

- Get a stand-up desk. You will burn 60 more calories per hour of standing at your computer than you do when sitting in front of it.

- When you need to use the restroom, hoof it to the farthest facility in your workplace to force yourself to walk more.

**EXERCISE**

## How to Burn Off 5,400 Calories Watching TV

Researchers at the University of Tennessee say you can burn almost 150 calories by walking in place during the commercials of a 1-hour TV show (roughly 25 minutes of ads). Since Americans watch an average of 36 hours of TV per week, that can add up to 5,400 calories.

- Schedule noontime walking meetings with staff.

- Stand whenever you talk on the phone.

- Tap your foot. Studies show that people who fidget tend to be thinner.

- Set your smart phone to remind you to take a rejuvenating walking break every hour.

- Three times a day, walk up three flights of stairs.

# READ 'EM AND REAP

Start on the five boosters above right away. Start today, even before you embark on your chosen Belly Off! Back-in-Shape Workout. Which you will begin tomorrow, right?

Your first day of the exercise plan will already put you ahead of most of your fellow Americans, fitnesswise. Recent surveys have shown that only about 33 percent of adults get any regular exercise. That's a very scary statistic. These folks are missing out on so many free health benefits that they would gain simply by taking the daily walk we prescribe on page 21. But those are benefits you'll be cashing in on, starting from day one. And they are benefits you can put a price tag on. Research in the *American Journal of Health Promotion* shows that people who are 30 to 60 pounds over their ideal weight spend $450 more on medical expenses per year than normal-weight people do. Men who lost 60 to 100 pounds, studies suggest, could save over $1,000 annually on doctor bills. Could you use an extra grand this year?

By making fitness a part of your life, you will reap many, many more rewards. Here's a look at what you can expect to gain from following the workout programs in this book.

**You'll drop pounds.** Exercising burns more calories than sitting on a couch with your face in a bowl of candy corn does.

# Recognize How Good Fitness Can Feel

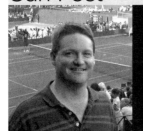

| Weight Before |
|---|
| **233** |

| Weight After |
|---|
| **185** |

## JEFF ATWATER
HUDSON, MA
THE BELLY OFF! CLUB, SEPTEMBER 2011

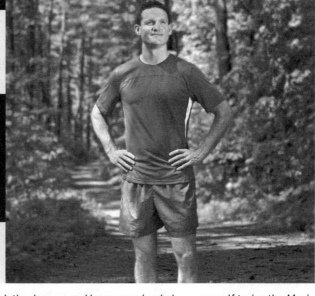

### THE WAKE-UP CALL

It wasn't an epiphany, but an opportunity. I'd wanted to lose weight and improve my health for a long time. Then one day I heard about a program called Belly Off! starting at a nearby gym. I signed up and read *The Belly Off! Diet.* We started with simple bodyweight exercises. They weren't easy, but after the workouts I really felt great. It was that good tiredness and feeling of satisfaction that comes over your body after exercising. That motivated me. I wanted more of that. Well, the program kickstarted a journey that found me weighing in at 185 pounds during my physical in December of 2010. Although the drop in the number on the scale has been fun to see, what is more important is that my strength, endurance, and physical health (including other health stats, such as cholesterol) have improved. I'm in better shape now at age 40 than I was in my late 20s and early 30s!

### HOW I CHANGED

I recognized the difference between feeling bloated from scarfing a pizza and soda and feeling comfortably full from eating foods containing fiber and protein. Building meals and snacks from whole grains and protein helped me cut out highly processed refined foods and beverages loaded with high-fructose corn syrup. Don't get me wrong—I still enjoy snacks and desserts like ice cream (I like Breyer's—especially vanilla, with its short, easily understood list of ingredients), but I usually make smarter choices of more filling foods like almonds or Greek yogurt with low-sugar granola. Another key change spurred by Belly Off! was that strength, conditioning, and cardio training became a regular part of my life. It was fun to rediscover how good regular activity makes me feel. I started adding weights to my bodyweight workouts. I found myself trying the *Men's Health* poster series workouts and 15-minute metabolic workouts. It was fun to try different things and challenge myself.

### THE REWARD

I trained for and ran the Seacoast Half Marathon twice, and then when I turned 40 I ran the Boston Marathon with the Dana-Farber Marathon Challenge team in support of cancer research. It was absolutely one of the most amazing experiences of my life. The crowds of people cheering you on; it was incredible. Fitness now, for me—well, it's part of my life. It's part of who I am.

## WEIGHT LOSS
## Mind Over Mac Attack

To stop thinking about going to the drive-thru, start thinking about going for a run in the park. According to the journal *Appetite*, mental imagery can reduce your desire to binge on food. When people in a study imagined themselves engaged in their favorite activities, their cravings were less intense.

How many more calories? Well, if you don't eat any fake corn, your body burns about 80 calories while watching an hour-long TV show. But go out for a walk for an hour, instead, and you'll burn about 320 calories. Not bad.

But don't forget that even after you've finished exercising, your metabolism stays elevated. That doesn't happen on the couch. If you've done high-intensity interval exercise, your calorie-burning fire may stay stoked for up to 42 hours. That means that if you're exercising almost every day, your metabolism is basically always running high. What's more, after a few weeks, when you've built new muscle through exercise, you'll be burning more calories all day and night because muscle requires more energy just to exist on your skeleton than fat does.

**You'll reduce your risk of diabetes.** As a result of losing weight and shedding your belly, you will reduce the amount of visceral fat surrounding your organs—a major risk factor for type 2 diabetes and heart disease. A new study by Harvard University researchers found that combining resistance training (weight lifting) with aerobic activity for a total of 300 minutes over the course of a week can reduce your risk of type 2 diabetes by up to 59 percent.

**You'll boost your energy.** Exercise strengthens that all-important muscle inside your chest—your heart. A lighter body puts less stress on your heart. A lighter body moves more efficiently and nimbly. When your heart and blood vessels aren't working so hard to pump oxygen and nutrients throughout all your limbs, you feel more energetic and empowered to keep going at work and during workouts. Your exercise routines will naturally become more rigorous, and your endurance will skyrocket. In addition, all of this will help you sleep more restfully and deeply. Recently, a study in the journal *Hypertension* demonstrated just how recuperative deep sleep can be. In a sleep study, scientists monitored the slow-wave sleep of a group of men. This is

**THE BELLY OFF! WORKOUTS**

## Food Diary

**Date:**

| | FOOD/DRINKS & AMOUNTS | FIBER | CALORIES |
|---|---|---|---|
| **BREAKFAST** | | | |
| **MORNING SNACK** | | | |
| **LUNCH** | | | |
| **AFTERNOON SNACK** | | | |
| **DINNER** | | | |
| **EVENING SNACK (OPTIONAL)** | | | |
| | | **TOTAL FIBER :** | **TOTAL CALORIES :** |

the deep, dreamless sleep that it is difficult to wake from. Those subjects who recorded the most slow-wave sleep were 45 percent less likely to develop high blood pressure than those who logged the least. The researchers say that this deep, recuperative sleep triggers brain signals that improve blood vessel flexibility.

**You'll be less stressed.** Physical activity releases feel-good endorphins that relieve stress, and it takes very little exercise to reap the benefit. A Scottish study of 20,000 adults found that working out for just 20 minutes a week helped lower stress and anxiety while increasing energy and happiness. Other studies

## Step Up to Go Down

Obese adults are six times more likely to lose weight if they weigh themselves at least once a week, according to a study in the *American Journal of Preventive Medicine*.

show that exercise can have a significant antidepressant effect. European researchers exploring the phenomenon believe they've found out why. It seems that intense exercise causes your adrenal glands to release the stress hormone cortisol into your bloodstream. In response, your blood activates a molecule called anandamide, which signals regions of your brain to release a substance called brain-derived neurotrophic factor, or BDNF. Too much of a science lesson? All you really need to know is that researchers say this substance, triggered by exercise, protects neurons from damage and acts as an antidepressant.

**You'll have better sex.** Exercise increases sexual arousal in both men and women. When you're fit, you feel better about your body and have more energy for sex. And men who are fit are at lower risk for developing erectile dysfunction.

**You'll think more clearly.** When you exercise, your heart feeds oxygen-rich blood to your brain, nourishing your gray matter. Researchers tracked 1,324 people involved in an aging study at the Mayo Clinic. They discovered that people who exercised

## A Jump-Start Safety Note
### FROM DAVID JACK

If you follow the advice in this book, in just 6 weeks you can expect to see a 15 to 20 percent improvement in your strength and cardiovascular output, as well as significant body fat loss. Most of these early gains will result from improved nutrition, drinking fewer liquid calories, moving more, and making better lifestyle choices. *The Belly Off! Workouts* strength-training component builds and preserves lean muscle tissue, reigniting your metabolism and burning more calories. Exercise is always accompanied by some risk, and this is especially true with strength training. There are three keys to managing risk.

1. Assess your ability and readiness for training. (See the self-screening tests in the appendix.)

2. Schedule a doctor's checkup to get a clean bill of health before embarking on any new fitness routine. You can raise any problems revealed in your self-screen at that time.

3. When training, be mentally present. Every rep. Don't daydream or get sidetracked by long conversation. Stay "in the workout." It'll produce a safer training environment and faster improvements.

moderately at age 50 and older were less likely to develop mild cognitive impairment later in life.

**You'll improve your immune function.** Experts say that even a short brisk walk 5 days a week can deliver a bigger boost to your immune system than eating oranges and green vegetables.

**You'll live longer.** It makes sense that all of these benefits of exercise would also translate to a longer, more active life. More and more research is proving the big impact exercise has on reducing disease and even fighting it when it strikes. Here's one example from a study at the University of Michigan: Researchers there examined the muscles of people with an advanced skin cancer. They found that those subjects with stronger, denser muscle tissue were 45 percent less likely to die of the deadly form of skin cancer than those who had less muscle. The researchers say that dense muscle is a reliable sign of better overall health and, perhaps, a stronger immune system.

Another study of more than 5,000 people found that those over age 50 who were highly physically active lived an average of 3½ years longer than those who were sedentary. And you can bet that they lived better, happier, more actively, and more energetically in their later years. All told, not a bad payback for getting back in shape with the Belly Off! Workouts.

**IT WORKS FOR ME**

Putting a spotlight on your fitness goals and diet details can help motivate you to keep on keeping on. That's what Belly Off! Club member Joe Lopez did. "I've started a fitness blog where I can post goals," he says. You'll be less likely to fall off a workout or nutrition program if you share your progress with the world. Try Word-Press or Posterous to start a fitness blog, or join the Belly Off! Club online at men-shealth.com/bellyoff. That's where you can post a profile and share your ups and downs with other members.

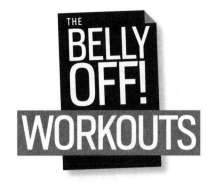

# Chapter 2

# MOVE MORE

## Begin Here with the Belly Off! Kick–Start Walking Program and Reap Health Benefits with Your First Step

Remember Newton's First Law from high school science class? "A body at rest tends to stay at rest . . . *eat too many brownies, and get fat*"? (Okay, maybe we edited that one a little!)

It's true—Sir Isaac's Law of Inertia applies to becoming overweight, too. A body in a constant state of rest—a sedentary body that doesn't move much—doesn't increase calorie

## Build Your Abs While You Walk

A high-intensity interval walking workout will shrink your belly far better than crunches, but you can tone your abs while frying calories by drawing your belly button toward your spine as you walk. Don't hold your breath, but do hold the contraction. You'll feel it working.

burn, doesn't fill its lungs with energizing oxygen, and tends to eat high-calorie foods from deep bowls in front of the television set. A body that stays at rest puts on extra weight and risks the dangers of obesity, diabetes, heart disease, and more.

Newton also said that an object will stay at rest unless an unbalanced force acts upon it. Well, consider this chapter your personal unbalanced force, a kick in the pants to start your body in motion.

We're not through with the science lessons, either. Consider these recent studies that spotlight the health benefits of moving your body—benefits that you'll gain with the first step.

**Shrink at least an inch from your waist.** Twenty minutes a day of brisk walking can help you reduce your waist size by at least 1 inch in 4 weeks, according to a review of 40 studies by the National Institutes of Health.

**Lose pounds without dieting.** A study at the University of Virginia compared people who walked at a leisurely pace 5 days a week with those who did three shorter, fast-paced walks and two longer, moderate-speed walks per week. While both groups burned the same 400 calories per workout, the people who exercised at a high intensity lost five times more fat from their midsections than the slow-walking group. The benefits didn't end there. The fast walkers also:

- Lost an average of more than 2 inches from their waistlines

- Shed three times more fat from their thighs

- Reduced dangerous visceral fat around the organs of their torsos

- Dropped nearly 8 pounds in 16 weeks through exercise alone, without dieting.

**Beat stress and anxiety.** Numerous studies have proven the feel-good benefits of exercise. It can combat depression, improve self-esteem, and stimulate relaxation. Walking research, in particular, shows that 20 to 30 minutes of brisk walking can trigger calming effects similar to those of a tranquilizer.

**Reduce risk of disease and death.** Reports in a 2012 issue of the medical journal *The Lancet* claimed that 9 percent of premature mortality—or more than 5.3 million deaths globally—in 2008 were due to physical inactivity. Researchers claim that even modest levels of activity, such as 15 to 30 minutes of brisk walking, bring significant health benefits.

Walking is a beautifully simple way to move more. It's the perfect exercise because it's easy and effective. Almost anyone can do it anywhere. It requires nothing but a comfortable pair of shoes and a little gumption. Walking is low-impact cardio, which makes it ideal for people who are overweight. For all of these reasons and more, we've made walking part of the Belly Off! Back-in-Shape Workouts, whether you choose the beginner, intermediate, or advanced sequence. Walking is simply *that* important to overall health, fitness, and weight maintenance.

On the following pages, you'll find two ways to start. Select the one that's recommended for your current level of fitness.

# THE 14-DAY WALKING KICK START

If you're overweight, have been sedentary for some months, are an absolute beginner, or feel that you need to start slower, the 14-Day Walking Kick Start is the perfect prelude to our 6-Week Back-in-Shape Workouts. You will do 2 weeks of daily walks designed to gradually increase your endurance and strength so that you will be ready for the beginner strength workout and the interval walking program, which is where your weight-loss afterburners will really kick in.

**EXERCISE**
## Walk This Way (to Burn More Calories)

Get your upper body into the action. Bend your elbows at 90 degrees and pump your arms as you walk. Doing so will automatically increase your pace, plus it will help you burn up to 15 percent more calories during each walking workout.

**FAT FACT**
## 86

Percentage of Americans who could end up overweight or obese, if current diet and fitness trends continue.

**EXERCISE**

## Put Your Intervals on Autopilot

Choosing a hilly, undulating walking or running route is a great way to create a natural interval workout.

■ **When going uphill,** look straight ahead, not at your feet. Keep your chest up and shoulders back; no hunching over.

■ **When going downhill,** look straight ahead, not at your feet; keep your torso upright and your nose over your toes; and control your steps so your feet don't slap the ground.

**WORKOUT 411**

*Note:* Beginners should complete this *before* starting the Belly Off! Beginner Back-in-Shape Workout.

■ Print out a calendar for the current month and stick it at eye level on your fridge or in another spot that you visit every day. Record how many minutes you walk every day, and use the calendar to ensure that you don't skip any walks.

■ Wear comfortable walking shoes or sneakers and loose-fitting clothing.

■ Walk with a friend, as long as he or she can keep up with your planned pace and won't slow you down. What kind of pace? Not a leisurely stroll, but a walk with purpose that's still easy enough that you can carry on a conversation while you move.

■ On days 6, 9, 12, and 14 pick up the pace to a power walk, which means you're going fast enough that you can speak only in short sentences. Eventually we'll move up to a jog, but we're getting ahead of ourselves.

■ Wear a watch or carry a cell phone so you can keep track of time. If the day's walk is 12 minutes, walk out for 6 minutes, then turn around and walk back. Or choose a circular route that you can finish in the allotted time.

■ Begin each walk slowly and work up to your pace. After the first 2 minutes, stop and do a few ankle rolls, shoulder rolls, reach-to-the-sky stretching, or anything else that feels right to loosen up your muscles. Then resume your workout pace.

■ After your walk, cool down by walking slowly for a minute or so and doing a few easy stretches.

# Belly Off! 14-Day Walking Kick Start Schedule

| DAY | 1 | 2 | 3 | 4 | 5 | 6 | 7 |
|---|---|---|---|---|---|---|---|
| TIME + PACE | 12 minutes, moderate | 12 minutes, moderate | 15 minutes, moderate | 18 minutes, moderate | 21 minutes, moderate | 15 minutes, brisk * | 23 minutes, moderate |

| DAY | 8 | 9 | 10 | 11 | 12 | 13 | 14 |
|---|---|---|---|---|---|---|---|
| TIME + PACE | 25 minutes, moderate | 18 minutes, brisk | 25 minutes, moderate | 28 minutes, moderate | 12 minutes, fast** | 30 minutes, moderate | 16 minutes, interval style *** |

\* Can speak only in short sentences
\*\* Difficult to speak in complete sentences
\*\*\* Starting and ending with an easy pace, alternate between moderate and brisk pace for 2-minute intervals

Once you finish your 2-week kick start, begin the Belly Off! Beginner Back-in-Shape Workout and the walking interval program described below.

# THE BELLY OFF! BACK-IN-SHAPE WALKING PROGRAM

It has been proven over and over again: Alternating between short bursts of moderate and high-intensity exercise burns more calories than steady-pace exercise does. Researchers at the University of Guelph in Ontario explain that pushing your body to intense activity levels boosts the ability of your cells to burn more fat. And by dialing back the intensity for a brief stint, your body gets a bit of rest so it can go intense again. What's more, because intervals force your body to work harder and faster, it takes longer for your metabolism to return to normal. That means your calorie burn stays elevated even after you've finished exercising. A study at the College of New Jersey found that men and women who did intervals burned about 15 percent more calories for about

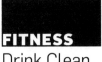

**FITNESS**
Drink Clean

Skip the sports drinks—they just add unwanted calories. Instead, drink water. It's all you need, even for your endurance walk.

**WEIGHT LOSS**

## 720 Seconds

**Walk for at least 12 minutes.** Studies show that you need at least that much activity at moderate to high intensity levels (where you are breathing somewhat hard) to reap the greatest fat loss. That level of activity boosts your body's ability to use oxygen and generate more of the fat-burning enzyme lipase, which breaks down fats.

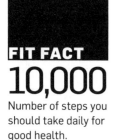

**FIT FACT**

# 10,000

Number of steps you should take daily for good health.

# 5,117

Average number of steps an American takes daily.

30 minutes after a workout than those who exercised at a moderate, steady pace.

- Start the Walking Intervals Program during Week 1 of any level of the Belly Off! Back-in-Shape Workouts.

- Warm up first. Why? Consider this: For every degree that your body temperature rises, the metabolic rate inside your cells increases by about 13 percent. Warm up by starting your walk at an easy to moderate pace for 3 to 5 minutes. That'll be long enough to push blood to your working muscles, raise your core temperature, and boost the activity of your fat-burning enzymes.

- Do interval-style walks three times a week.

- Do two 20- or 30-minute steady-pace walks at a moderate pace per week.

- Go long once a week. Despite our enthusiasm for intervals, there's still a benefit to doing an occasional endurance workout. So once a week, go for a long walk—at least an hour. Constant movement for 60 minutes at a moderate pace will force your body to dip into its fuel reserves, giving you yet another fat-burning metabolic lift.

**Extra Credit:** During Week 2, try pushing yourself harder on interval days by adding metabolism-revving calisthenics to the mix. See "40-Minute Interval Super Fat Burn (Plus Calisthenics)" on page 26.

# Weeks 1 and 2

| Monday | Tuesday | Wednesday | Thursday | Friday | Saturday | Sunday |
|---|---|---|---|---|---|---|
| 30-Minute Interval Walk (below) | 20-Minute Steady Moderate Walk | 30-Minute Interval Walk (below) | 30-Minute Steady Moderate Walk | 30-Minute Interval Walk (below) | 60-Minute Endurance Walk | 20-Minute Steady Moderate Walk |

# 30-Minute Interval Walk

| TIME | PACE | INTENSITY* |
|---|---|---|
| 5 minutes | Warmup | 3 |
| 3 minutes | Moderate | 5 or 6 |
| 2 minutes | Brisk | 7 or 8 |
| 2 minutes | Fast | 9 |
| 2 minutes | Moderate | 5 or 6 |
| 2 minutes | Fast | 9 |
| 2 minutes | Moderate | 5 or 6 |
| 2 minutes | Fast | 9 |
| 2 minutes | Moderate | 5 or 6 |
| 2 minutes | Fast | 9 |
| 2 minutes | Moderate | 5 or 6 |
| 2 minutes | Brisk | 7 or 8 |
| 2 minutes | Cooldown | 3 |

*On a scale of 1 to 10, with 1 through 4 meaning it's easy to speak normally, 5 and 6 meaning it's challenging to speak in long sentences without trouble, 7 and 8 meaning you're breathing harder and can only speak in very short sentences, and 9 and 10 meaning you can't speak because you're too busy gasping for breath.

## EXERCISE
### Take Time

If you go out without a watch, you're going to have to guesstimate your intervals. Instead, wear a sports watch and use the interval function. Or use your smartphone. You can download the free app Gymboss 2 Interval Timer from the iTunes app store. Customize your interval length and it will sound a tone when it's time to switch pace.

# Weeks 3 and 4

| Monday | Tuesday | Wednesday | Thursday | Friday | Saturday | Sunday |
|---|---|---|---|---|---|---|
| 40-Minute Interval Super Fat Burn (Plus Calisthenics) (below) | 30-Minute Steady Moderate Walk | 40-Minute Interval Super Fat Burn (Plus Calisthenics) (below) | 30-Minute Steady Moderate Walk | 40-Minute Interval Super Fat Burn (Plus Calisthenics) (below) | 60-Minute Endurance Walk | 20-Minute Steady Moderate Walk |

# 40-Minute Interval Super Fat Burn (Plus Calisthenics)

| TIME | PACE | INTENSITY* |
|---|---|---|
| 3 minutes | Warmup | 3, increasing to 6 |
| 3 minutes | Moderate | 5 or 6 |
| 2 minutes | Brisk | 7 or 8 |
| 2 minutes | Fast | 9 |
| 2 minutes | Brisk | 7 or 8 |
| 2 minutes | Moderate | 5 or 6 |
| 30 seconds | Jumping jacks | |
| 2 minutes | Moderate | 5 or 6 |
| 2 minutes | Brisk | 7 or 8 |
| 2 minutes | Fast | 9 |
| 30 seconds | Feet together, side-to-side hops | |
| 2 minutes | Moderate | 5 or 6 |
| 2 minutes | Brisk | 7 or 8 |
| 1 minute | Fast | 9 |
| 30 seconds | Jumping jacks | |
| 2 minutes | Moderate | 5 or 6 |
| 2 minutes | Brisk | 7 or 8 |
| 2 minutes | Fast | 9 |
| 30 seconds | Feet together, side-to-side hops | |
| 1 minute | Moderate | 5 or 6 |
| 1 minute | Brisk | 7 or 8 |
| 1 minute | Fast | 9 |
| 3 minutes | Cooldown | |

*On a scale of 1 to 10, with 1 through 4 meaning it's easy to speak normally, 5 and 6 meaning it's challenging to speak in long sentences without trouble, 7 and 8 meaning you're breathing harder and can only speak in very short sentences, and 9 and 10 meaning you can't speak because you're too busy gasping for breath.

Weeks 5 and 6 include steady-state walks, walking intervals, endurance walks, and walk/run intervals, with the goal of building up to 30 minutes of slow running.

# Week 5

| Monday | Tuesday | Wednesday | Thursday | Friday | Saturday | Sunday |
|---|---|---|---|---|---|---|
| 30-Minute Interval Walk/Run (walk for 2 minutes, run for 1 minute; repeat 10 times; walk for 3 minutes to cool down) | 30-Minute Steady Moderate Walk | 40-Minute Interval Super Fat Burn (Plus Calisthenics) | 30-Minute Steady Moderate Walk | 30-Minute Interval Walk/Run (walk for 1 minute, run for 4 minutes; repeat 6 times; walk for 3 minutes to cool down) | 60-Minute Endurance Walk | 20-Minute Steady Moderate Walk |

# Week 6

| Monday | Tuesday | Wednesday | Thursday | Friday | Saturday | Sunday |
|---|---|---|---|---|---|---|
| 30-Minute Interval Walk/Run (walk for 1 minute, run for 5 minutes; repeat 5 times; walk for 3 minutes to cool down) | 30-Minute Steady Moderate Walk | 30-Minute Interval Walk/Run (walk for 1 minute, run for 9 minutes; repeat 3 times; walk for 3 minutes to cool down) | 30-Minute Steady Moderate Walk | 35-Minute Interval Walk/Run (walk for 1 minute, run for 5 minutes, walk for 1 minute, run for 10 minutes, walk for 1 minute, run for 15 minutes, walk for 2 minutes; walk for 3 minutes to cool down) | 30-Minute Run (at an easy pace; walk for 3 minutes to cool down) | 30-Minute Steady Moderate Walk |

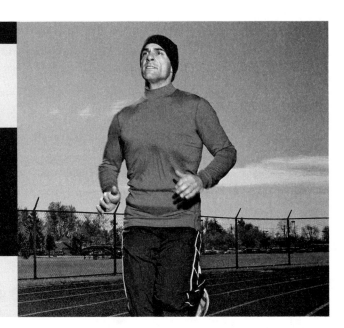

# Never Play Hooky from Workouts

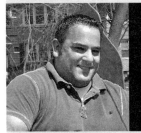

**Weight Before**

# 286

**Weight After**

# 163

## RICH VITTORIA

BUFFALO, NY
THE BELLY OFF! CLUB, JANUARY 2010

### THE WAKE-UP CALL

I'm a fourth-grade teacher whose students never gave him apples. They knew what I liked: cupcakes, brownies, and cookies. Those snacks were a great perk of the job, but then I met a better one: my future wife, Sarah. She's an apple-loving girl, and when I asked her to marry me, I resolved to shape up. So I dropped nearly 50 pounds. But I slipped up after our wedding, and my bingeing grew worse after our sons were born. I ballooned to nearly 300 pounds.

Forget being able to play with my sons—I was afraid I wouldn't even see them grow up. My blood pressure skyrocketed. Then I was diagnosed with sleep apnea, which forced me to sleep with a mask connected to a machine that blew air into my windpipe to keep it open. The first time I wore it, my 3-year-old son was afraid to say good night to me. That's when I realized it was time to lose the weight for good.

### HOW I CHANGED

The day I started exercising, I set out to run a mile—and made it past about six houses. But I wasn't discouraged. I just tried to run a little farther each time. As my stamina increased, I started weight training. I also work my core by doing side planks for as long as I can hold them. Most important, I never skip a workout. Since I don't play hooky from work, I figure there's no reason to play hooky from exercising.

My diet is another story. I started by paring down my plate. I measured my food and learned that my "normal" portions (like a half pound of pasta) were anything but. I don't eat out as much anymore, but when I do, I look at nutrition info online and decide beforehand what I'll eat. I'm also the family cook, and I load up our meals with vegetables. Instead of buying lunch at work, I pack one, like tuna on a wrap plus some celery and peanut butter. I still have my sweet tooth, but that's okay: If you deprive yourself of desserts entirely, you'll go insane.

### THE REWARD

My sleep apnea has disappeared, and I no longer need the machine. I shed 14 inches from my waist. Finally, I look and feel like the professional teacher I am. But even better than that, I'm a role model for my sons and students. My students bring carrots and other healthful foods for their snacks. As these kids grow up, I know they'll think fitness and healthy eating are as essential as doing homework. It's the best lesson I've ever taught them.

# Chapter 3

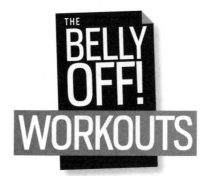

# THE NEW BELLY OFF! 2-MINUTE DRILL

## A No-Excuses, Total-Body-Wake-Up Call. Do It Daily.

What are you doing tomorrow morning before stumbling into the kitchen? Got a couple of minutes? That's all it takes to get your blood pumping and jump-start your fat-burning metabolism.

The Belly Off! 2-Minute Drill is an ideal way to wake up and start your day on a positive health note.

It involves eight easy, heart rate–boosting exercises. Crank them out before you eat breakfast or take a shower. They require just 120 seconds of your time: about as long as it takes to brush your teeth. In this chapter, we'll show you three different versions—beginner, intermediate, and advanced. Choose the one best suited to you and progress to the more challenging drills over time.

Get in the habit of doing the Belly Off! 2-Minute Drill every morning. It'll be a daily reminder to move your body more throughout the day. In fact, you may want to repeat the 2-Minute Drill as a midmorning jolt in place of a coffee break, a lunchtime heart-pounder, or a 3 p.m. clear-the-cobwebs drill that can be done anywhere, even at work. On the busiest of days, when you just can't devote time to the regular workouts in this book, snag a few 2-minute windows of free time to accumulate enough 2-minute drills, along with a brisk walk, to reach that 30-minute daily fitness quota that ensures good health.

The 2-Minute Drill also makes for a perfect warmup for the resistance and interval training workouts in this book or any other sports activity because it engages the 10 common physical skills required for sports performance and a healthy, active life: strength, cardiovascular endurance, stamina, flexibility, power, speed, coordination, accuracy, agility, and balance.

## A DYNAMIC, TOTAL-BODY WARMUP

Most people warm up with a few minutes on a treadmill followed by some static stretching. Well, that's simply not good enough. It addresses very few of the skill sets we mentioned above, and it doesn't adequately increase your heart rate. The Belly Off! 2-Minute Drill offers all of that in a single functional-training warmup that can be done anywhere, using only your body weight. (No gear!)

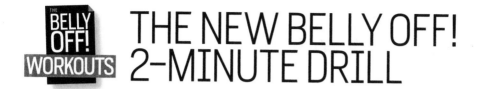

# THE NEW BELLY OFF! 2-MINUTE DRILL

## BEGINNER

Do the drill at half-speed, meaning at a moderate effort level of 5 on a scale where 1 is slow motion and 10 is all-out. If you choose to do a second or third round in the morning or to string several together for a workout increase your effort level with each round: a 7 or 8 effort level for round 2; a 9 or 10 effort level for round 3. Don't sacrifice form for speed.

## DO EVERY MORNING

# BEGINNER 2-MINUTE DRILL PUNCH LIST

Do each exercise for 15 seconds. For moves 1, 3, and 7, switch positions roughly halfway through and try to complete an equal number of reps per side.

1. Arm Circle, Forward and Backward
2. March in Place
3. Step Forward, Step Backward
4. Cow and Cat
5. T Hinge
6. Glute Bridge
7. Bird Dog
8. Jumping Jack

**(cut and tape to your bathroom mirror)**

# ARM CIRCLE, FORWARD AND BACKWARD

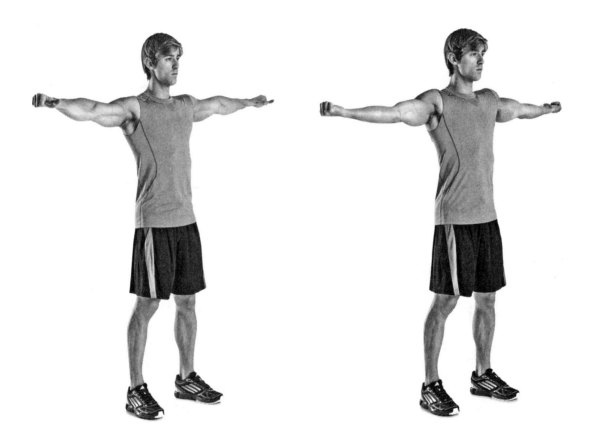

Standing tall, raise your arms out to your sides so that they are parallel with the floor. Point your thumbs forward. Using your shoulders and upper back, create small, tight circles with your arms. Keep your shoulders down and your chin and neck in line with your body. Halfway though the 15 seconds (about 15 quick circles), rotate your thumbs so they point backward. Make small backward circles for the remainder of the 15 seconds.

# MARCH IN PLACE

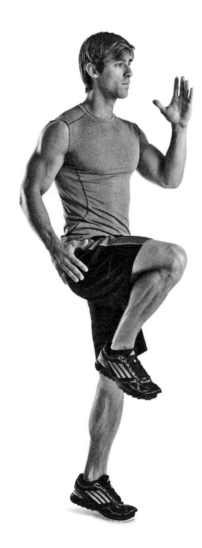

Stand tall and march in a diligent yet relaxed fashion. Bend your arms
and swing them as you march, bringing your hands to about chin height with
each swing. This sounds easy, but focus on good form, driving your legs
and feet down through the floor for 15 seconds to get your blood pumping.

# STEP FORWARD, STEP BACKWARD

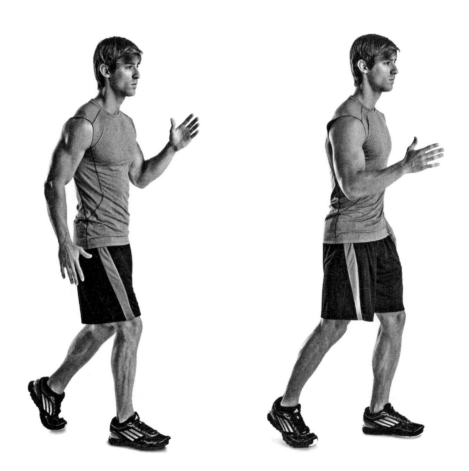

With feet hip-width apart, step forward with your right leg as if to begin walking, but stop yourself by landing on the ball of your foot, bending your left knee, and dropping your hip slightly. Pause and immediately drive your right foot through the ground to push your body backward so that your right leg stops behind your body, leaving you in a similar high lunge position, right leg bent, ball of your right foot on the floor. Pause and repeat for half of the 15 seconds (3 to 5 reps). Switch sides to lead with your left leg for the remainder of the 15 seconds. Focus on taking deliberate steps and on your balance.

# COW AND CAT

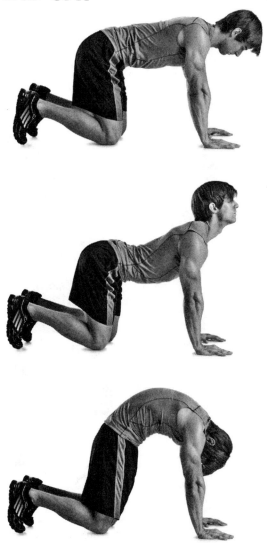

This two-part move engages your abs and stretches your upper and lower back and shoulders. Get on all fours, with your knees under your hips and your hands under your shoulders. Exhale as you slightly push your belly button toward the ground to create a small arch in your low back (avoid this move if you have back trouble). Then inhale as you pull your belly button up into your spine and bow your back as much as possible, as if mimicking a cat stretch. Repeat as many times as you can in 15 seconds.

# T HINGE

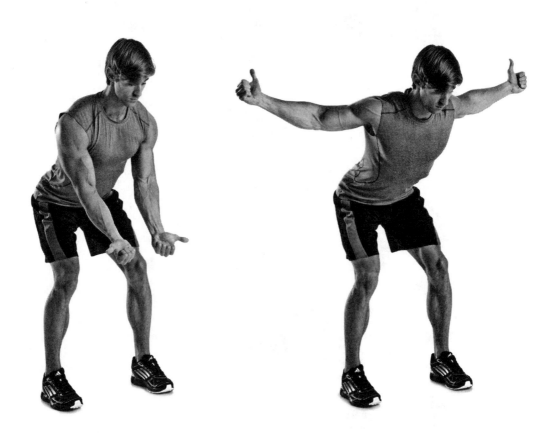

Stand with your feet shoulder-width apart. Unlock your knees and push
your hips backward as you lower your upper body, creating a stretch in the
backs of your legs. Be sure to put weight into your hips and heels. Hold
your arms in front of you, palms up, thumbs pointing out. Drive your arms
out and away from your body, with your thumbs pointing backward.
Squeeze your shoulder blades together as you open your chest. Then,
return your arms to center and stand by squeezing your glutes to push
your hips forward and driving your knees backward. Do as many as you
can in 15 seconds.

# GLUTE BRIDGE

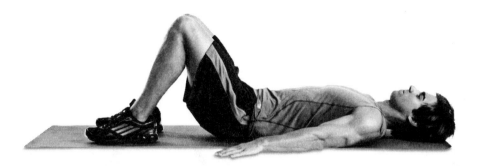

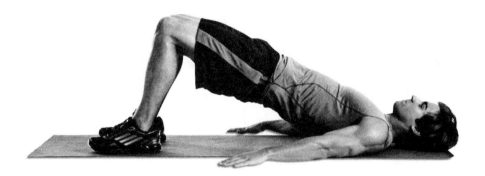

Lie on your back with your arms out to your sides, palms down, knees bent, and feet flat on the floor. Press your feet into the floor and squeeze your glutes to raise your hips up and back so that your body forms a straight line from your shoulders to your knees. Keep your head on the floor and do not arch your back. Pause at the top and squeeze your glutes as hard as you can, lower your body to the floor, and repeat for 15 seconds.

# BIRD DOG

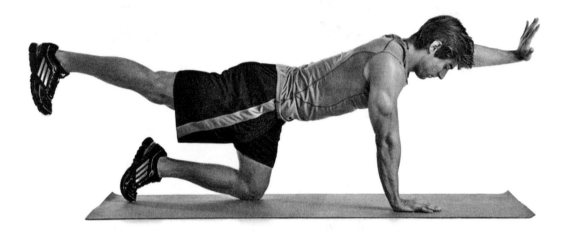

Get on all fours, with your knees under your hips and your hands under your shoulders. Keeping your neck and spine in line, extend your right leg out straight behind you while simultaneously extending your left arm straight ahead, holding both parallel with the floor. Pause and return to the starting position. Repeat with your opposite leg and arm, alternating for 15 seconds. Minimize the arch in your back and keep your body from swaying or moving as you raise and lower your arms and legs. Great for stretching and strengthening your lower back.

# JUMPING JACK

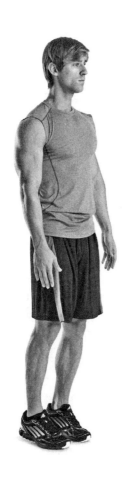
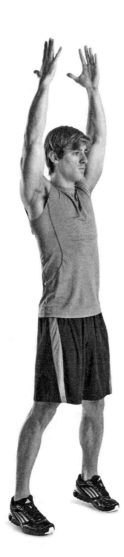

Stand with your feet hip-width apart and your arms at your sides. Drive your arms overhead as you simultaneously jump and separate your feet to the sides, then immediately jump back to the starting position. Keep a slight bend in your knees, and your weight on the balls of your feet throughout the exercise. Repeat for 15 seconds.

# INTERMEDIATE

The intermediate 2-minute drill is a progression from the beginner drill, incorporating more challenging moves requiring greater strength, balance, and endurance. Do this 2-minute drill at half-speed, meaning at a moderate effort level of 5 on a scale where 1 is slow motion and 10 is all-out. If you choose to do a second or third round in the morning or to string several together for a workout warmup, increase your effort level with each round: a 7 or 8 effort level for round 2; a 9 or 10 for round 3.

## DO EVERY MORNING

# INTERMEDIATE 2-MINUTE DRILL PUNCH LIST

Do each exercise for 15 seconds. For moves 1, 3, 6, and 7, switch positions roughly halfway through and try to complete an equal number of reps per side.

1. Arm Circle, Forward and Backward, with Balance
2. Skip, with Arm Swing
3. Step Backward with Trunk Rotation
4. Skater Hop (with Tap)
5. Pushup Plank to Down Dog
6. Glute Bridge with March
7. Power Squat
8. High Knee Run in Place

**(cut and tape to your bathroom mirror)**

# ARM CIRCLE, FORWARD AND BACKWARD, WITH BALANCE

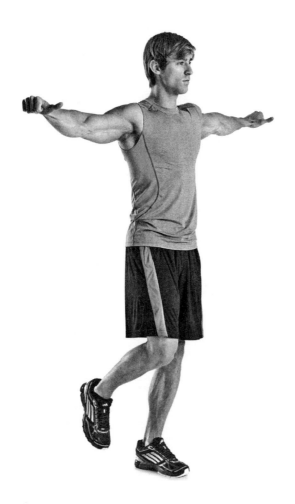

Perform the alternating forward and backward arm circles as described on page 32 while balancing on one foot. Rotate your arms backward 3 times, switch feet to balance on your opposite foot, and rotate your arms forward 3 times. Continue alternating legs and arm circle direction for the 15 seconds. Focus on making small, tight arm-circle patterns. If you lose your balance, tap one foot on the ground to gain control and restart the movement.

# SKIP, WITH ARM SWING

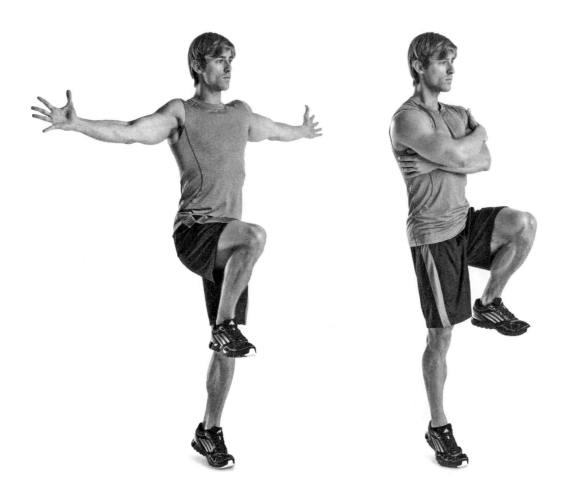

Skip just as you did when you were a kid, but lift your arms up so
they're parallel with the floor and swing them out and away from your
body and then back across your body, as if you're giving yourself a bear
a hug with every skip. Repeat for 15 seconds.

# STEP BACKWARD WITH TRUNK ROTATION

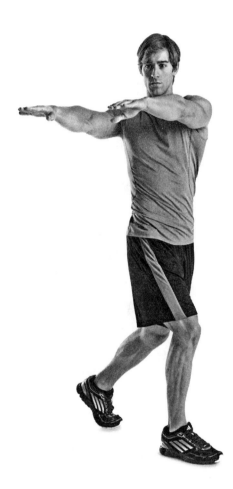

With your arms held straight out in front of you, parallel to the floor, step backward with your left leg so the ball of your left foot is on the ground behind you. Bend your right leg and keep your right foot flat on the ground. Keep your chest up. Rotate your arms and upper trunk to the right, across your forward leg. Rotate back to the center position and step up. Repeat the move, this time stepping back with your right leg and rotating your extended arms to the left, across your left leg. Repeat for 15 seconds.

# SKATER HOP (WITH TAP)

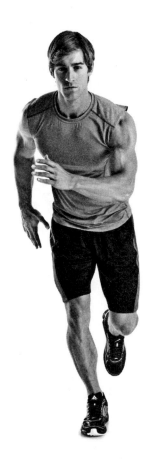
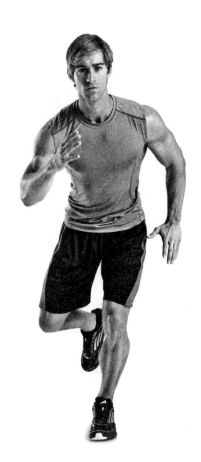

Crouch over your right foot and lift your left leg off the floor behind you. Bound to your left by pushing off with your right leg. Land on your left foot, lifting your right leg off the floor behind you. Continue hopping back and forth. Tap your foot behind you for balance; make small, controlled hops to start. Repeat for 15 seconds.

# PUSHUP PLANK TO DOWN DOG

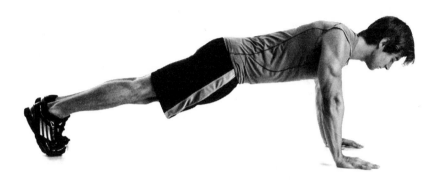

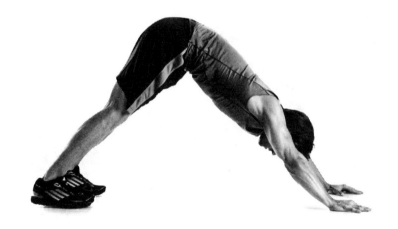

Get into a pushup position, with your arms straight under your shoulders. Now, drive your hips up and back by pushing your arms through the ground and pulling your belly button up into your spine. You should end up in yoga's Down Dog position, an upside-down V with your butt at the apex. Try to keep the heels of your feet as close to the ground as possible, maintain a flat back, and relax your head between your arms. Pause and return quickly to the top pushup position by dropping your hips. Stop the downward momentum of your body by engaging your core, hips, legs, and arms. Repeat for 15 seconds. You can add a full pushup in between to increase the difficulty.

# GLUTE BRIDGE WITH MARCH

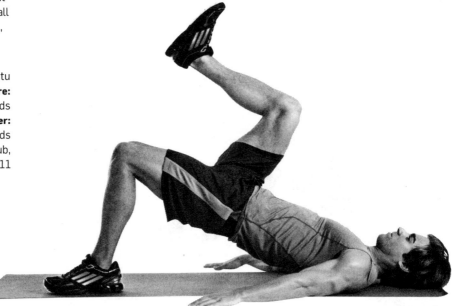

Lie on your back with your arms out to your sides and resting on the floor, knees bent, and feet flat on the floor. Press your feet into the floor and squeeze your glutes to raise your hips up and back so that your body forms a straight line from your shoulders to your knees. Keep your head on the floor and do not arch your back. Pause at the top and squeeze your glutes as hard as you can. Once you have set this position (or found your home base, as we call it), raise one leg off the floor toward your chest by bending your knee, and then lower it back to the floor. Repeat with the opposite leg. Continue alternating leg lifts while maintaining a good bridge for 15 seconds.

# POWER SQUAT

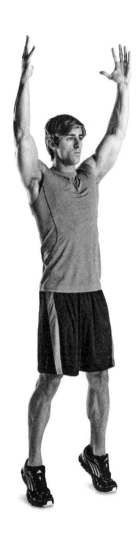

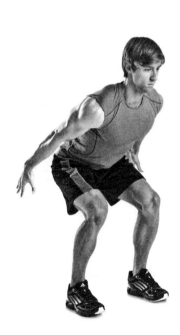

Stand tall, with your feet spread a bit wider than hip-width apart, and raise both arms above your head as you rise up on your toes. Balance for a second, and then drive your hands aggressively down and back past your hips as you quickly lower into a squat position with your feet flat on the ground, hips back, chest up, and knees over your ankles (not caving in). Pause for 1 second and then drive your body back up onto your toes by swinging your arms overhead. Repeat for 15 seconds.

# HIGH KNEE RUN IN PLACE

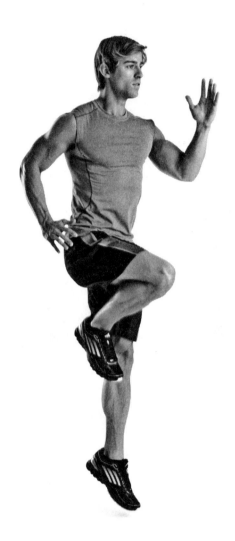

Run in place, lifting each knee high as you would while running in tall grass or about a foot of water. Drive your arms up and down and back aggressively as you pump your legs. Stay on the balls of your feet, and keep your chest up and eyes forward. Run as fast as you can for 15 seconds, imagining that the floor is red-hot and you want to get your feet off of it as quickly as possible.

## ADVANCED

The advanced 2-minute drill contains more challenging and aggressive progressions to the intermediate version. Do the 2-minute drill at half-speed, meaning at a moderate effort level of 5 on a scale where 1 is slow motion and 10 is all-out. If you choose to do a second or third round in the morning or to string several together for a workout warmup, increase your effort level with each round: a 7 or 8 effort level for round 2; a 9 or 10 for round 3.

## DO EVERY MORNING

# ADVANCED 2-MINUTE DRILL PUNCH LIST

Do each exercise for 15 seconds. For moves 2 and 4, switch positions roughly halfway through and try to complete an equal number of reps per side.

1. Split Squat Switch with Arm Circle Forward and Backward
2. Step Backward to Skip
3. Crab Reach
4. Glute Bridge with Leg Swing
5. Reverse Pushup
6. Skater Hop with Arm Drive
7. Squat Jump
8. Wall Drive

(cut and tape to your bathroom mirror)

# SPLIT SQUAT SWITCH WITH ARM CIRCLE FORWARD AND BACKWARD

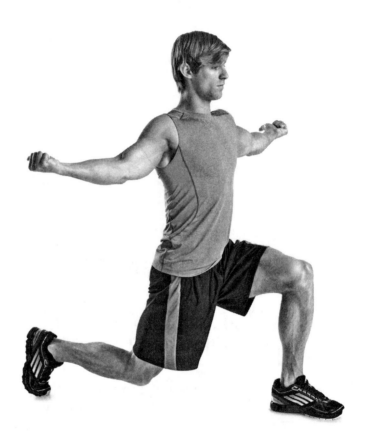

Begin in a tall split squat stance with your left leg in front, knee slightly bent, foot flat, and your trailing leg (right) behind you on the ball of your foot. Extend your arms out to your sides and parallel with the floor. Circle your arms forward (holding your thumbs backward as well) 3 times, and then jump to switch foot positions—right foot forward, left foot back—and circle your arms in the reverse direction. The circles should be small, as if your hands were tracing the rim of a salad plate. Continue to alternate quickly for 15 seconds.

# STEP BACKWARD TO SKIP

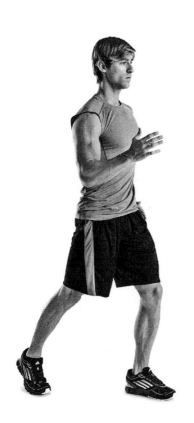
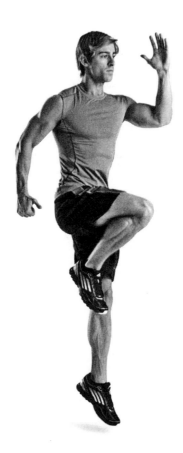

From a standing position with your feet hip-width apart, step backward
with your right leg into a reverse lunge position so the ball of your right foot
is on the ground behind you. Bend your left leg and keep your left foot flat
on the ground. Pause, and then explode up into a skip, driving your right
knee up and swinging your arms forward as you skip up and off the ground,
land, and return to the step back position. Transition quickly and repeat
on one side for half of the time. Switch sides for the remainder of the
15 seconds.

# CRAB REACH

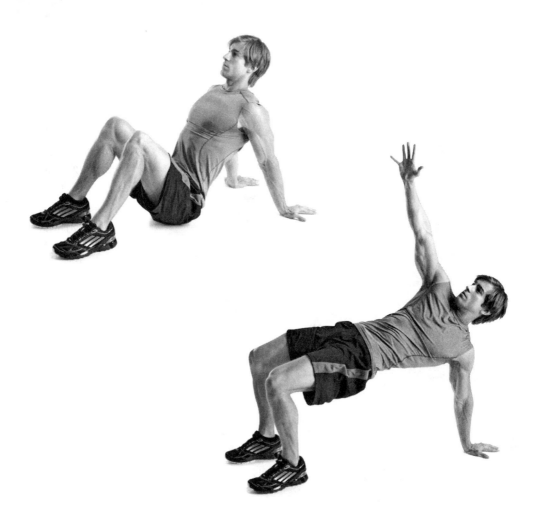

Assume a "crab" position: chest facing the ceiling, hands and feet flat on the floor, arms straight under your shoulders, and knees bent. Keep your back flat, chest open, and head in line with your body. That's the starting position. Drive your hips up and reach your right hand toward the ceiling. Your supporting arm and legs and your core should be engaged to support your reaching arm. Return your right arm and body to the starting position and repeat the move using your left arm. Continue alternating arms for 15 seconds.

# GLUTE BRIDGE WITH LEG SWING

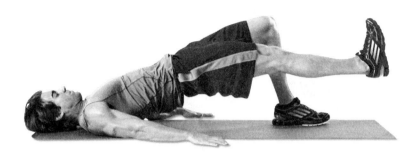

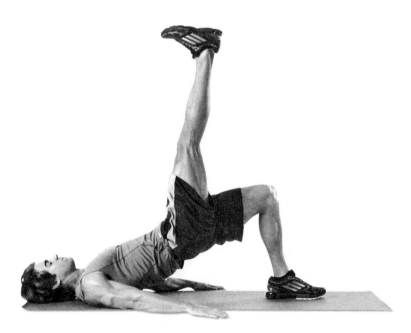

Lie on your back with your arms out to your sides and resting on the floor, knees bent, and feet flat on the floor. Press your feet into the floor and squeeze your glutes to raise your hips up and back so that your body forms a straight line from your shoulders to your knees. Keep your head on the floor and do not arch your back. Pause at the top and squeeze your glutes as hard as you can. Once you have set this position (or found your home base, as we call it), extend your right leg straight out. Now swing it up toward the ceiling and back down to the straight out position. Halfway through the 15 seconds, switch to your left leg and repeat.

# REVERSE PUSHUP

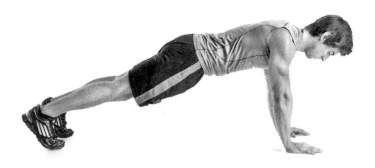

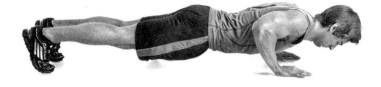

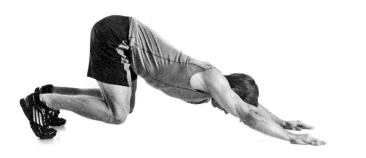

Assume a pushup position, with your arms straight and hands slightly wider than shoulder-width apart. Bend your elbows and lower your torso until your chest nearly touches the floor. Pause, and then straighten your arms as you push your butt toward your ankles until your knees are bent at 90 degrees. Return to the starting position and repeat for 15 seconds.

# SKATER HOP WITH ARM DRIVE

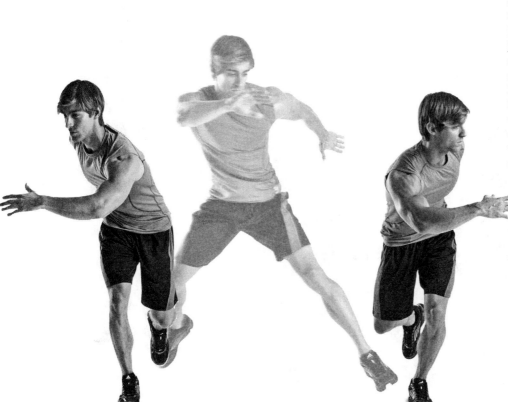

Crouch over your right foot and lift your left leg off the floor behind you. Bound to your left by pushing off with your right leg. Land on your left foot, lifting your right leg off the floor behind you. Continue hopping back and forth for 15 seconds. You can tap your foot behind you for balance; otherwise, try to keep your lifted foot off the floor. Drive your right arm vigorously to your left across your body when hopping left, and drive your left arm right when hopping right.

# SQUAT JUMP

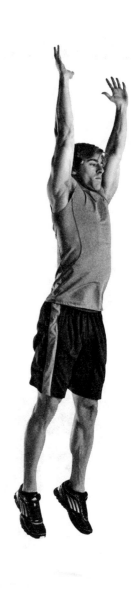
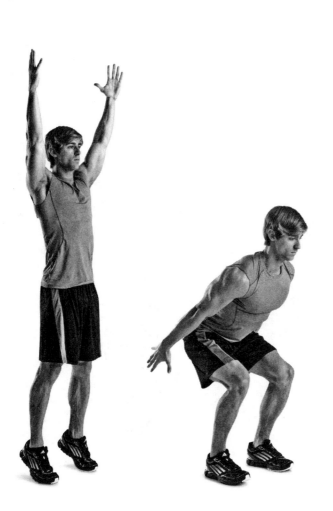

Stand tall, with your feet spread a bit wider than shoulder-width apart, toes forward, and hands above your head. Simultaneously push your hips back and swing your arms down to your sides, lowering your body until your thighs are nearly parallel to the floor. Explode up forcefully so your feet leave the ground. Repeat for 15 seconds.

# WALL DRIVE

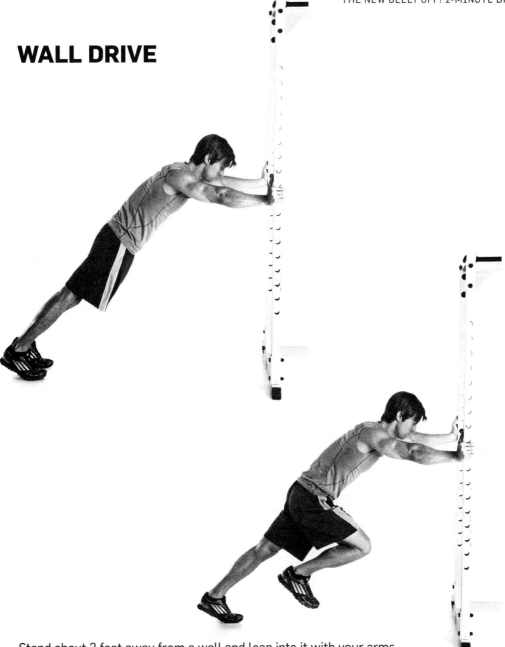

Stand about 3 feet away from a wall and lean into it with your arms straight and parallel to the floor. Your body should lean toward the wall at about a 45-degree angle. Bend your right knee and lift your right leg until your thigh is parallel to the floor or higher. Do a high-knee run for 15 seconds by switching leg positions explosively as you push into the wall. Drive the trailing leg through the ground as the lead knee moves forward.

# PART

# 2

## BACK-IN-SHAPE WORKOUTS

Why is it that so many of us lousy golfers always come back to play again?

It's because no matter how frustrating the game is, we love it. It's fun. And no matter how poorly a round we may play, we always hit a couple memorable Rory McIlroy–like shots that give us profound joy—and hope that maybe, just maybe, we're starting to improve. That's what keeps us coming back.

Even if you've never played, you can learn something from golf that can be applied to exercise and workouts: You need to keep yourself coming back for more, even when you're frustrated and tired and feeling more like a duffer than a pro.

The secret to sticking with exercise is similar to what turns people passionate about golf:

a) It must be fun.

b) It must give you hope.

Exercise can't be a drag or you won't be able to drag yourself to do it for more than a week. And it must induce optimism by delivering results quickly. We humans need positive feedback to avoid discouragement (and to avoid breaking $400 graphite golf clubs over our knees). That's why we recommend logging your workouts and recording the number of reps and the time it takes to complete your sets. As the weeks go by, you will be encouraged by the gains illustrated by your workout log.

Many members of the Belly Off! Club have told us that the importance of these two criteria—fun and feedback—is among the greatest lessons they've learned along their journey. So please make sure to choose exercise you enjoy, and remember to savor the little wins.

The Belly Off! workouts were built with that in mind. We want them to be fun and challenging, with built-in progressions so you can easily see and feel them working.

In the following chapters, you'll find three workout programs, one designed for beginners, an intermediate progression, and an advanced workout. You decide where you'd like to begin.

If you haven't exercised in a long while or you are 20 or more pounds overweight, the beginner workout is an excellent place to start. In fact, it's not a bad place to start no matter what kind of shape you're in. It virtually ensures that you won't injure yourself by going too hard, too fast, as the workout is designed to establish core strength and stability. Then, after you've finished the 6-week program, move on to the intermediate workout, and then to the advanced.

THE BELLY OFF! WORKOUTS

Chapter 4

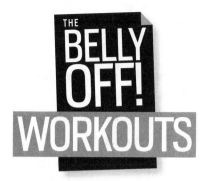

# THE BELLY OFF! BEGINNER BACK-IN-SHAPE WORKOUT

## Your Launching Pad to Amazing Results!

You're going to love this workout because it's quick and easy and it delivers fast improvement to goose your motivation. This program centers on several key movement patterns that will forge a foundation of fitness you can build upon. You'll burn fat, develop cardiovascular endurance, build muscle and strength, patterns that begin to establish healthy lifestyle habits for life.

■ The Beginner Back-in-Shape Workout assumes that you have completed the Belly Off! 14-Day Walking Kick Start or you are already a walker or runner.

■ Perform three strength workout sessions each week, and walk every day, using the Belly Off! Back-in-Shape Walking Program starting on page 23. If three workouts are too much for you, do two for the first 2 weeks, then increase to three once the initial muscle soreness eases.

■ Warmup with either the Beginner 2-Minute Drill at 50 to 60 percent effort or 3 to 5 minutes of any light cardio exercise.

■ After your warmup, perform the Belly Off! Flex Series stretches (starting on the opposite page). Important: As tempted as you'll be to dive right into the strength workout, do not skip these brief warmups, which will prepare your body for work and protect you from injury.

■ Alternate between Strength Workout A and Workout B, resting for a day in between workouts. There are a total of five exercises in each. The first three moves are included in both workouts. Do 1 set of each. The last two resistance exercises change between workouts A and B. You will do 5 sets each of these final two moves.

■ Cool down with another round of either the Flex Series stretches or 3 minutes of walking. Your choice. Ideally, you should do both if you have the time.

# BELLY OFF! FLEX SERIES

Do this after your 2-minute drill as part of your cardio warmup. These dynamic moves are designed to prepare your muscles and central nervous system for the workouts that follow. Warm, prepared muscles will perform better and resist injury better than cold muscles. Do 1 set in the following order.

## WRIST ROLL
### FORWARD AND BACK, 10 REPS EACH WAY

Extend your arms up and away from your body at a 45-degree angle to the floor. Keeping your arms stationary, make circles with your hands by flexing your wrists. Be sure to relax your entire hands, including your fingers. Do 10, then reverse the direction and do 10 more.

## SHOULDER ROLL
### FORWARD AND BACK, 10 REPS EACH WAY

Stand tall and place your hands in front of your body, near the tops of your thighs. Letting your elbows bend slightly, roll your shoulders in big circles backward, bringing them up toward your ears and then back and away from you while trying to open your chest. Do 10, then reverse the direction and do 10 more.

## HIP CIRCLE
### 5 REPS EACH LEG

Place the palms of your hands against a wall in front of you. Walk your feet back a few steps so that you are leaning slightly into the wall, bending at your ankles, not at your waist. Pick your right foot and knee up and out, as if you were stepping over a track field hurdle, while keeping your body tall and your left foot rooted into the ground. Don't force the hurdle step—try to lift smoothly while allowing your right hip to open slightly outward as you step up and over. Perform 5 reps with your right leg, then switch sides and repeat.

**GET JACKED!**

Resistance bands are some of the most versatile exercise tools you can own. They are portable and inexpensive, and you can do hundreds of exercises with them. Unlike weights, resistance bands create constant tension throughout a resistance movement, recruiting more muscle fibers and accelerating growth.

—David Jack

# ANKLE CIRCLE
## 10 REPS EACH FOOT

Stand on one foot (use a wall, railing, or chair back for support if needed, but try to keep your balance without it), lifting your other foot slightly off the ground in front of you. Keeping your leg stationary, draw 10 large, smooth circles in one direction with your toes pointed. Lower your leg and repeat the exercise using your right foot.

# TWIST AND PRESS
## 10 REPS

Stand with your feet slightly wider than shoulder-width apart and your arms at your sides, elbows bent at 90-degree angles. With a relaxed, flowing motion, rotate your torso and hips toward your left while driving your right arm out in the same direction, as if pushing an object away from you. (Think of it like a karate palm strike). Lift your right heel and pivot on the ball of that foot to allow your hips to move with your torso. Once your right arm is fully extended, immediately twist to your right, pulling your right hand back toward your rib cage and driving your left arm toward your right. The motion should be fluid, and your head, chest, and belly button should move together as a unit as the foot of your trailing leg rotates to allow your hips to follow your upper body.

# SINGLE LEG THREE-WAY STEP
## 5 REPS EACH LEG

For this move, you will balance on one leg as you reach the other out to tap the ground at three different points: directly in front of you, to the side, and behind. Begin by balancing on your right foot. Bend at your hips and right knee, as if you are beginning to sit down into a chair, and reach your left foot forward as far as you can under control and lightly touch the floor with your heel. Return to standing straight up, then bend at your hips and right knee again to reach and tap your left heel at the 9 o'clock position. Return your leg to center, then reach your left foot behind you while rotating your torso and hips left slightly to bend and touch your heel at about the 7 o'clock position. Try to keep your right knee from traveling forward of your foot. That's 1 repetition. Repeat 4 more times, then do 5 reps on the opposite side.

# STANDING QUAD STRETCH (WALL SUPPORTED)
## 6 REPS EACH LEG

Stand facing a wall, and place your left hand on the wall for support. Grab the front of your right ankle with your right hand, bend your knee, and pull your heel toward your backside. Keep your knee under your body; don't let it pull out to the side. Hold that position for 2 seconds while pushing your hips toward the wall by squeezing your glutes, not by arching your back. Release your foot to the floor. That's 1 repetition. Repeat the stretch 5 more times with the same leg, then do 6 reps on the opposite leg.

# ISOMETRIC DOORWAY SPREAD APART
## 5 REPS

Stand about 1 foot in front of an open doorway with your feet shoulder-width apart, your knees slightly bent, and your chest up. Place the outsides of your forearms at about rib height on each doorjamb, palms facing one another. Use your back and shoulders to pull your arms open, as if trying to spread the door apart with your forearms. Use about 60 percent of your total effort. Hold this position for 5 seconds, then relax and repeat 4 more times. Do not shrug your shoulders during this move.

# ISOMETRIC DOORWAY CHEST FLY
## 5 REPS

Stand in a doorway with your back close to one side of the doorjam, your feet shoulder-width apart, and your chest up. With your knees slightly bent, extend your arms parallel to the floor and elbows slightly bent and place the palms of your hands on opposite sides of the door frame (or walls, if your arms are long). Squeeze your hands toward each other and into the walls by squeezing your pectorals together. Hold for 5 seconds, then release and repeat.

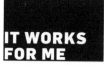

**IT WORKS FOR ME**

"Get a friend to take on the weight-loss challenge with you. I did, and now I have the attitude that I can't quit because he's not going to."

—Matt Deiss
**Weight Before:**
279 pounds
**Weight After:**
190 pounds
The Belly Off! Club,
May 2002

# THE 6-WEEK BEGINNER STRENGTH WORKOUT

There are three resistance workouts each week (either A or B is repeated, as indicated below). Always rest for at least 1 day between resistance workouts. You will walk every day, including on your Workout A and B days, using the Belly Off! Walking Program explained on page 23.

## Week 1

| MONDAY | TUESDAY | WEDNESDAY | THURSDAY | FRIDAY | SATURDAY | SUNDAY |
|---|---|---|---|---|---|---|
| Strength Workout A / 30-Minute Interval Walk | Rest* / 20-Minute Steady Moderate Walk | Strength Workout B / 30-Minute Interval Walk | Rest / 30-Minute Steady Moderate Walk | Strength Workout A / 30-Minute Interval Walk | 60-Minute Endurance Walk | 20-Minute Steady Moderate Walk |

* Always rest for 1 day between strength workouts, but continue with daily walking.

## Week 2

| MONDAY | TUESDAY | WEDNESDAY | THURSDAY | FRIDAY | SATURDAY | SUNDAY |
|---|---|---|---|---|---|---|
| Strength Workout B / 30-Minute Interval Walk | Rest* / 20-Minute Steady Moderate Walk | Strength Workout A / 30-Minute Interval Walk | Rest / 30-Minute Steady Moderate Walk | Strength Workout B / 30-Minute Interval Walk | 60-Minute Endurance Walk | 20-Minute Steady Moderate Walk |

* Always rest for 1 day between strength workouts, but continue with daily walking.

# Strength Workout A

Workout A contains five exercises. The first three resistance moves—Reverse Lunge and Hold, Power Squat, and Lateral Skater Step and Tap—are repeated in Workout B. Do only 1 set of these exercises.

The last two resistance exercises differ between workouts. In Workout A, you will do Pushups and Box Squats, 5 sets of each move. The first set of pushups and box squats is called your "master set," which means you should do as many repetitions as you can with good form and without rest, until you start to feel a burn or your form suffers. But don't do more than 20 reps total.

Rest for 1 to 2 minutes before starting the next set. For the remaining 4 sets, perform half the number of reps you completed in your master set, resting as needed between sets. Once you've finished all 5 sets of pushups, move on to your box squats. (Option: If you find that you are too fatigued to do all sets of one exercise back-to-back, you may alternate between the last two exercises—the pushups and box squat—in this five-move series. Either way, expect to feel sore the day after this workout! Never push yourself to muscle failure on any repetition.) Record the number of reps in your master sets as well as the length of time it took to complete Workout A, so you can track your progress.

# WEEKS 1 TO 2

## WORKOUT A

### WARMUP

Beginner 2-Minute Drill (see page 31)
Flex Series (see page 63)

| STRENGTH EXERCISES | REPS | SETS |
|---|---|---|
| REVERSE LUNGE AND HOLD | 5 (each leg) | 1 |
| POWER SQUAT | 10 | 1 |
| LATERAL SKATER STEP AND TAP | 8 (each way) | 1 |
| PUSHUP | Master set | 1 |
| | ½ master set | 4 |
| BOX SQUAT | Master set | 1 |
| | ½ master set | 4 |

## COOLDOWN

Walk (3 minutes)
Flex Series (see page 63)

# REVERSE LUNGE AND HOLD

**MUSCLE**
## Stretch for Strength

A study at Brigham Young University–Hawaii found that beginning lifters who did static stretching on their nontraining days grew stronger than lifters who didn't stretch. Researchers say that lengthening muscle fibers through stretching causes them to allow faster contraction speeds, which can result in increased power.

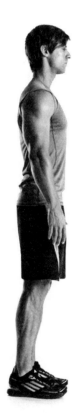

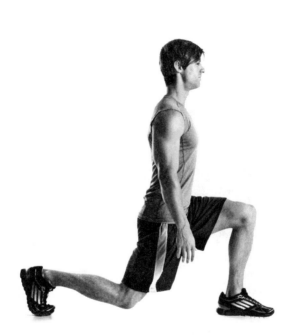

Stand with your legs shoulder-width apart. Take a step backward with your right foot and lower yourself down into a lunge position. (Work toward a goal of having your right knee almost touch the ground and your left thigh be parallel to the ground.) Keep your back straight and make sure your left knee doesn't extend past your toes. Balance in this position for 3 seconds, then return to standing. Do 4 more on the same leg, then repeat on the opposite leg.

# POWER SQUAT

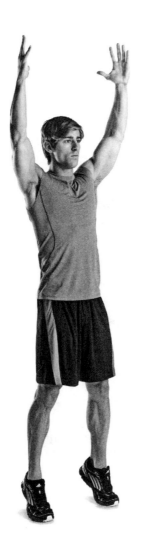

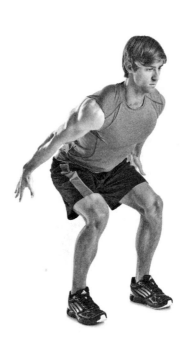

Stand with your feet slightly more than shoulder-width apart, toes forward, hands stretched up and above your head. Simultaneously push your hips back and drive your arms down to your sides, lowering your body until your thighs are nearly parallel to the floor. Hold for 4 seconds, and then explode up to the starting position without allowing your feet to leave the floor. Repeat 9 more times.

# LATERAL SKATER STEP AND TAP

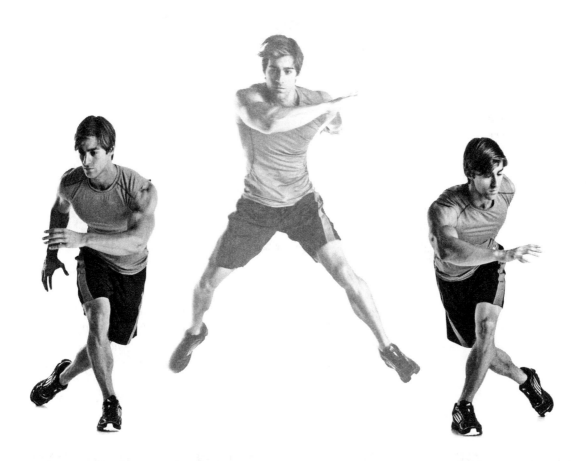

Stand with your feet hip-width apart, knees and arms slightly bent, leaning forward a bit at your waist. Leap to the right at least 2 feet and allow your left foot to tap the floor behind and outside your right foot. Immediately bound back to the left, landing on your left foot and allowing your right foot to tap the floor behind and outside your left. This exercise is similar to a speed skater's side-to-side movement, and as such it should involve swinging your arms for momentum, your outside arm swinging in front of your body in the direction of your travel. Continue back and forth this way for 8 bounds to each side.

# PUSHUP

## Make Pushups Harder

You are pressing about 64 percent of your body weight during a standard pushup. Elevate your feet on a 2-foot-high exercise bench and you'll increase that to 74 percent.

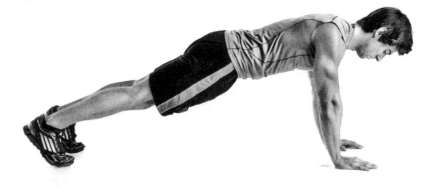

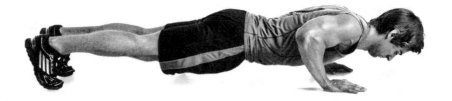

This classic exercise is ideal for strengthening your upper body. Support yourself with straight arms, placing your hands on the floor directly underneath your shoulders and your toes on the floor about hip-width apart. Your back should be straight from head to heels. Bend your arms to lower yourself to touch your chest to the floor. Keep your abdominal muscles taut by imagining that you're drawing your belly button toward your spine. Press yourself back to the starting position. Repeat.

## WHAT IF I CAN'T DO MANY PUSHUPS?

If you have difficulty doing 10 pushups with good form, that's okay. Do modified pushups until you've built up your chest and arm strength and lost some weight so you can complete 10 good ones.

Pushups become easier when you increase the angle of your body, and there are many ways to do this. Try doing pushups on your knees, rather than toes. Try them with your feet on the floor and your hands elevated on a sturdy box or step. Still too hard? Place your hands on a park bench. We prefer wall pushups to

kneeling, because they build better core strength. Stand about 2 feet from a wall. Lean into the wall with your hands spread about shoulder-width apart and your arms straight. Lower your torso to the wall, then push yourself back. As you become stronger, gradually reduce the angle of your body by placing your hands on lower supports, which increases the resistance on your chest and arms. Work your way down to the ground, and get working on your master set.

# BOX SQUAT

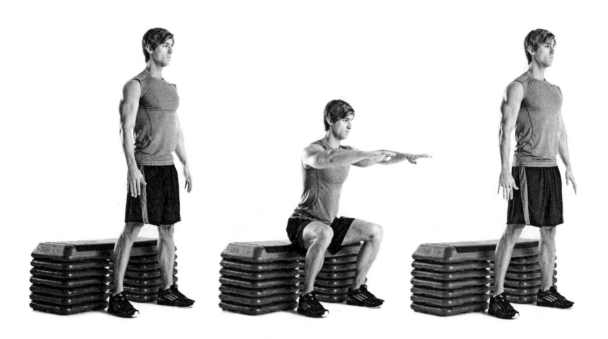

The box squat is a terrific exercise for learning proper squat technique because it ensures that you lower yourself to an adequate and safe depth and develop explosive strength. Start by finding a sturdy box or chair that's tall enough for your butt to touch it when your thighs are about parallel to the floor. Place your feet shoulder-width apart, toes pointing slightly out. With your core tight and arms out for balance, sit back toward the box by moving your hips back at the same time as you bend your knees. (This is called a bone rhythm movement, where you move two or more joints simultaneously; it's a technique that eliminates undue stress on your joints, such as the stress that can happen when you move only, say, your hips or your knees.) Keeping your chest up and core engaged throughout the exercise, use a controlled movement to descend as far as you can or until you lightly touch the box with your butt. Never bounce off the box or chair. Pause for a second and, keeping your weight on your heels and in the balls of your feet, drive your feet through the floor explosively to return to the standing position. Don't allow your back to bow.

**FIT FACT**

# 150

Number of calories
you can burn simply
by walking in place
during the commer-
cials of a 1-hour-long
TV show, according
to a University of
Tennessee study.

# Strength Workout B

As with Workout A, there are a total of five exercises in Workout
B. The first three are the same as in Workout A. Do only
1 set of each of these.

The new exercises in Workout B are the Split Squat and
Inverted Row. The first set of each is your "master set," which
means you should do as many repetitions as you can with good
form and without rest, until you start to feel a burn or your
form suffers. Don't do more than 20 reps total. Do your master
set of split squats with your dominant leg forward. You can
pencil your reps right into the chart on the opposite page.
For the remaining 4 sets, perform half the number of reps you
completed in your master set, resting as needed between sets.

For this pairing of new exercises, alternate between sets of
the split squat and the inverted row, switching leg positions for
each set of split squats. This will allow your legs to recover for
a set of rows instead of fatiguing from back-to-back squats. Rest
as needed between sets.

# WEEKS 1 TO 2

# WORKOUT B

## WARMUP

Beginner 2-Minute Drill (see page 31) + Flex Series (see page 63)

| STRENGTH EXERCISES | REPS | SETS |
|---|---|---|
| **REVERSE LUNGE AND HOLD** | 5 (each leg) | 1 |
| **POWER SQUAT** | 10 | 1 |
| **LATERAL SKATER STEP AND TAP** | 8 (each way) | 1 |
| **SPLIT SQUAT** | Master set | 1 |
| (dominant leg) | | |
| **INVERTED ROW*** | Master set | 1 |
| **SPLIT SQUAT** | ½ master set | 1 |
| (opposite leg) | | |
| **INVERTED ROW** | ½ master set | 1 |
| **SPLIT SQUAT** | ½ master set | 1 |
| (dominant leg) | | |
| **INVERTED ROW** | ½ master set | 1 |
| **SPLIT SQUAT** | ½ master set | 1 |
| (opposite leg) | | |
| **INVERTED ROW** | ½ master set | 1 |
| **SPLIT SQUAT** | ½ master set | 1 |
| (dominant leg) | | |
| **INVERTED ROW** | ½ master set | 1 |
| **SPLIT SQUAT** | ½ master set | 1 |
| (opposite leg) | | |

*Alternate exercise: Supported Single-Arm Dumbbell Row (each arm)

## COOLDOWN

Walk (3 minutes) + Flex Series (see page 63)

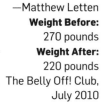
# SPLIT SQUAT

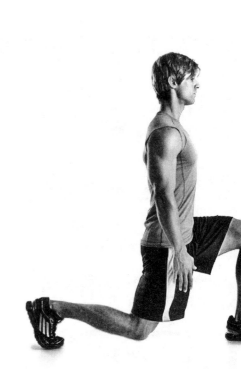

Stand in a staggered stance, your dominant foot flat on the floor in front of you and your other foot 2 to 3 feet behind, resting on the ball of your foot. Slowly lower your body as far as you can; your rear knee should nearly touch the floor. Your front shin should be nearly perpendicular to the ground, and your knee should stay right above your ankle, not lean inward or outward. Make sure your front heel stays on the ground. Keep your torso upright and your core engaged throughout the movement. Pause, then push yourself up to the starting position as quickly as you can.

# INVERTED ROW

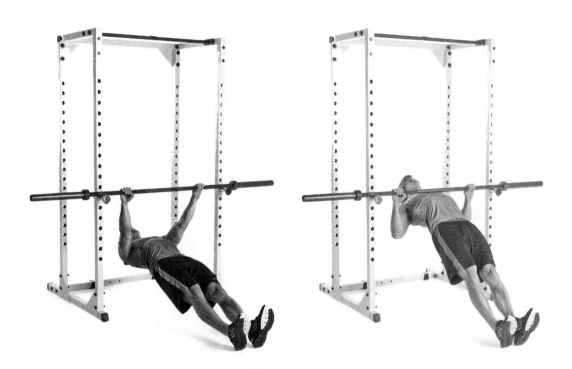

Mount a chinup bar in a doorway about 3 feet from the floor. (If you don't
have the gear to do an inverted row, substitute a Supported Single-Arm
Dumbbell Row, see page 78.) Lie faceup underneath the bar with your
heels on the floor, and grab the bar using an overhand grip, hands spaced
a bit more than shoulder-width apart. Keeping your body in a straight line
from heels to head, bend your arms and pull your chest to the bar, using
mostly your back muscles and squeezing your shoulder blades together
at the top of the movement. Slowly lower yourself until your arms are
straight. Repeat. *Note:* To increase the difficulty, you can lower the bar.
To make it easier, raise the bar, bend your knees, or split your feet (one foot
forward, one back) and use the back leg for support and assistance.
(Do not shrug your shoulders throughout the movement.)

# SUPPORTED SINGLE-ARM DUMBBELL ROW
## (ALTERNATIVE FOR INVERTED ROW)

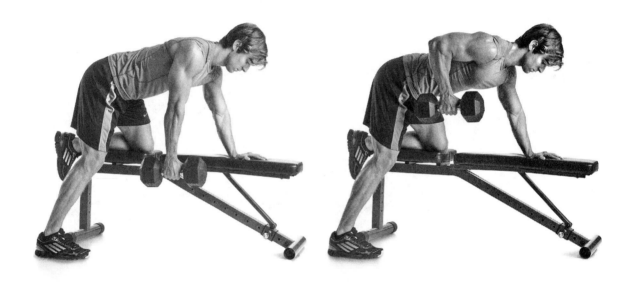

Grab a dumbbell in your right hand and place your left hand and left knee on a flat bench. Keep your back flat and your upper body parallel to the floor. Let your right arm hang straight down from your shoulder, with your palm facing inward toward the bench. Pull the dumbbell toward your rib cage until your right upper arm is just past parallel to the floor, with your elbow above your torso. Avoid curling your wrist and shrugging your shoulder as you become fatigued. Pause, lower, and repeat. After completing all reps on your right side, repeat the exercise on the opposite side.

# WEEKS 3 THROUGH 5

Now that you have established a foundation of conditioning, it's time to take it up a notch. You will increase the number of reps in each workout and, to boost your metabolic conditioning, you will add calisthenics (jumping jacks and high-knee runs) in between two of the strength exercises.

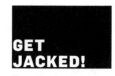

**GET JACKED!**

Exercise is great, but your early results will hinge on what you ate!

—David Jack

## DETERMINE YOUR MAX

The day before beginning your third week, determine your new "maximum set" (the max number of reps you can do in a continuous set until you lose good form) with each of the Week 3 through 5 strength exercises—pushup, power squat, inverted row, and split squat. This number will guide your workouts during Week 3. Retest your max set at the beginning of weeks 4 and 5, as well. Each new number will guide your workouts during those weeks.

## Week 3

| MONDAY | TUESDAY | WEDNESDAY | THURSDAY | FRIDAY | SATURDAY | SUNDAY |
|---|---|---|---|---|---|---|
| Strength Workout A / 40-Minute Super Fat Burn Walk | Rest*/ 30-Minute Steady Moderate Walk | Strength Workout B / 40-Minute Super Fat Burn Walk | Rest*/ 30-Minute Steady Moderate Walk | Strength Workout A / 40-Minute Super Fat Burn Walk | 60-Minute Endurance Walk | 20-Minute Steady Moderate Walk |

\* Always rest for 1 day between strength workouts, but continue with daily walking.

## Week 4

| MONDAY | TUESDAY | WEDNESDAY | THURSDAY | FRIDAY | SATURDAY | SUNDAY |
|---|---|---|---|---|---|---|
| Strength Workout B / 40-Minute Super Fat Burn Walk | Rest*/ 30-Minute Steady Moderate Walk | Strength Workout A / 40-Minute Super Fat Burn Walk | Rest*/ 30-Minute Steady Moderate Walk | Strength Workout B / 40-Minute Super Fat Burn Walk | 60-Minute Endurance Walk | 20-Minute Steady Moderate Walk |

\* Always rest for 1 day between strength workouts, but continue with daily walking.

# Week 5

| MONDAY | TUESDAY | WEDNESDAY | THURSDAY | FRIDAY | SATURDAY | SUNDAY |
|--------|---------|-----------|----------|--------|----------|--------|
| Strength Workout A / 30-Minute Interval Walk/Run (page 27) | Rest* / 30-Minute Steady Moderate Walk | Strength Workout B / 40-Minute Super Fat Burn Walk | Rest* / 30-Minute Steady Moderate Walk | Strength Workout A / 30-Minute Interval Walk/Run (page 27) | 60-Minute Endurance Walk | 20-Minute Steady Moderate Walk |

*Always rest for 1 day between strength workouts, but continue with daily walking.

# Strength Workout A with Calisthenics

Now that you have your max set number for each of these exercises, multiply that number by 3 to get the total number of reps you will do during your workout. For example, if the most pushups you can do straight through is 12, you would get 36 ($3 \times 12 = 36$). If you were able to do 20 power squats under control with good form, your total number of reps of squats for the workout would be 60 ($3 \times 20 = 60$). No matter what your max set is, do no more than a total of 60 pushups or 75 squats in one workout.

During this workout, alternate between the Pushup and the Power Squat. In between those strength moves, alternate between 20 reps of the Jumping Jack and 20 reps (each step counts) of the High-Knee Run.

Rest as needed between sets to manage your fatigue. Your goal is to perform each exercise with good form and complete the total number of reps using as many sets as you need. Tip: It will help to perform more reps in the sets at the beginning of your workout and decrease the number as you become more fatigued. Using the example above of 36 total pushups and 60 total power squats, your workout may look something like the chart on the opposite page.

# WEEKS 3 TO 5

# WORKOUT A

## WARMUP

Beginner 2-Minute Drill (see page 31)
Flex Series (see page 63)

| STRENGTH EXERCISES | REPS | CUMULATIVE REPS |
|---|---|---|
| PUSHUP | 12 | 12 |
| JUMPING JACK | 20 | |
| POWER SQUAT | 20 | 20 |
| HIGH-KNEE RUN | 20 | |
| PUSHUP | 10 | 22 |
| JUMPING JACK | 20 | |
| POWER SQUAT | 15 | 35 |
| HIGH-KNEE RUN | 20 | |
| PUSHUP | 8 | 30 |
| JUMPING JACK | 20 | |
| POWER SQUAT | 13 | 48 |
| HIGH-KNEE RUN | 20 | |
| PUSHUP | 6 | 36 total/done |
| JUMPING JACK | 20 | |
| POWER SQUAT | 12 | 60 total/done |
| HIGH-KNEE RUN | | |

**Record your total time and max set reps:** _____, _____, _____ *
(Time)          (Pushups)          (Power Squats)

* Make it your goal to improve your time with each new workout.

# COOLDOWN

Walk (3 minutes)
Flex Series (see page 63)

# Strength Workout B with Calisthenics

The flow for Weeks 3 to 5 Workout B is similar to that of Workout A, but instead of multiplying your max set by 3 for your inverted row, multiply by 4. If, for example, you can do a maximum of 10 inverted rows, 4 × 10 gives you 40 reps for a workout target. For the split squat, continue to multiply by 3. For example, if you can do a maximum of 20 alternating split squats, 3 × 20 gives you 60 reps for a workout target. In between the strength movies do calisthenics, alternating between the Side-to-Side Hop and Line Run. (Don't exceed 40 total inverted row reps or 60 split squats in your first workout.)

## CALISTHENICS
## SIDE-TO-SIDE HOP (TWO-FOOTED)

Stand with your feet hip-width apart. Hop about 1 foot to your right, landing with both feet on the floor simultaneously. Immediately hop 1 foot back to your left. (That's 2 reps.) Do 20 as rapidly as you can with good form. Maintain a slight knee bend throughout the movement.

## LINE RUN

Use chalk to draw a line on the pavement. Stand with both feet behind the line. Your goal is to move your feet back and forth over the line: Step forward with your right foot and follow with your left. As soon as the ball of your left foot hits the pavement across the line, step back over the line. Imagine that the floor is red-hot and you must lift your feet off the ground as quickly as you can. Stay on the balls of your feet and pump your arms as you run. Over and back with both feet equals 1 rep. Be smooth and quick, and lead with a different foot with each subsequent set.

# WEEKS 3 TO 5

# WORKOUT B

## WARMUP

Beginner 2-Minute Drill (see page 31)
Flex Series (see page 63)

| STRENGTH EXERCISES | REPS | CUMULATIVE REPS |
|---|:---:|:---:|
| INVERTED ROW | 10 | |
| SIDE-TO-SIDE HOP | 20 | |
| SPLIT SQUAT | 20 | |
| LINE RUN | 20 | |
| INVERTED ROW | 8 | 18 |
| SIDE-TO-SIDE HOP | 20 | |
| SPLIT SQUAT | 16 | 36 |
| LINE RUN | 20 | |
| INVERTED ROW | 8 | 26 |
| SIDE-TO-SIDE HOP | 20 | |
| SPLIT SQUAT | 14 | 50 |
| LINE RUN | 20 | |
| SPLIT SQUAT | 10 | 60 total/done |
| SIDE-TO-SIDE HOP | 20 | |
| INVERTED ROW | 6 | 40 total/done |

**Record your total time and max set reps:** _____, _____, _____ *
                                            (Time)           (Inverted Row)      (Split Squats)

*Make it your goal to improve your time with each new workout.

# COOLDOWN

Walk (3 minutes)
Flex Series (see page 63)

# WEEK 6

This week, we've created a larger circuit and added a greater cardiovascular element to the program to get you ready to transition to the Intermediate workout. The Week 6 workout uses a type of circuit known as MRT, or metabolic resistance training, because it's fast-paced and done with very little rest. It's pretty intense, designed to spike your metabolism and torch serious fat by combining aerobic and compound muscular training moves.

We call this week's workout Crazy 8 because it incorporates eight of the exercises you've used over the past 5 weeks, with a couple of crazy tweaks. You will do this workout three times during this final week, with a rest day between each one.

For each exercise, perform as many repetitions as possible, minus 1. That means leave 1 good rep in your tank by monitoring your fatigue level and stopping just 1 rep before your form would start to get sloppy—what trainers call "technique failure."

Circuits should be done with very little rest between individual exercises, but you may rest briefly as needed, attempting to complete the circuit as quickly as possible. Be sure to rest for up to 2 minutes in between completed circuits. You'll need it! Perform 2 Crazy 8 circuits on day 1. Perform 3 circuits on workout days 2 and 3 during this final week of the Beginner program.

## WHAT NOW?
## Next Steps on Your Belly Off! Journey

After completing Week 6 of the Beginner workout, you may choose to move on to the Intermediate body-weight workout beginning on page 92. Another option: Repeat the Week 6 Crazy 8 workout for a few more weeks while pushing yourself to complete the circuits faster and faster. Record how long it takes to complete 3 back-to-back circuits and try knocking seconds off your time with each subsequent workout. It's a great way to track your progress.

# Week 6

| MONDAY | TUESDAY | WEDNESDAY | THURSDAY | FRIDAY | SATURDAY | SUNDAY |
|--------|---------|-----------|----------|--------|----------|--------|
| Crazy 8 (2 circuits) / 30-Minute Interval Walk/Run (see page 27) | Rest* / 30-Minute Steady Moderate Walk | Crazy 8 (3 circuits) / 30-Minute Interval Walk/Run (see page 27) | Rest* / 30-Minute Steady Moderate Walk | Crazy 8 (3 circuits) / 35-Minute Interval Walk/Run (see page 27) | 30-Minute Easy-Pace Run | 30-Minute Steady Moderate Walk |

* Always rest for 1 day between strength workouts, but continue with daily walking.

# WEEK 6

# WORKOUT CRAZY 8
## WARMUP
Beginner 2-Minute Drill (see page 31)
Flex Series (see page 63)

| STRENGTH EXERCISES | REPS |
|--------------------|------|
| PUSHUP | As many as possible with good form minus 1 |
| JUMPING JACK | 20 |
| POWER SQUAT | As many as possible with good form minus 1 |
| HIGH-KNEE RUN | 20 |
| INVERTED ROW | As many as possible with good form minus 1 |
| SIDE-TO-SIDE HOP | 20 |
| REVERSE LUNGE (no hold; alternating legs) | As many as possible with good form minus 1 |
| LINE RUN | 20 |

**Record your total workout time:** _____ *

* Make it your goal to improve your time with each new workout.

# COOLDOWN
Walk (3 minutes)
Flex Series (see page 63)

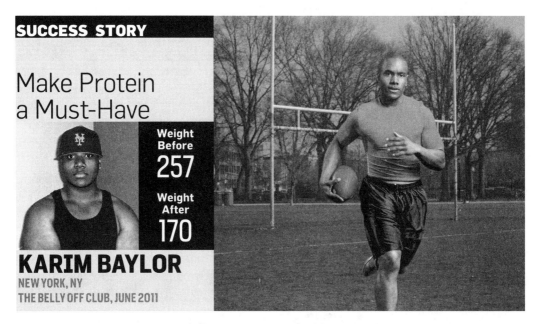

## SUCCESS STORY

# Make Protein a Must-Have

**Weight Before**
## 257

**Weight After**
## 170

## KARIM BAYLOR
NEW YORK, NY
THE BELLY OFF CLUB, JUNE 2011

### THE WAKE-UP CALL

I went to college in Miami, where I wanted to spend time on the beach with all the girls in bikinis—but man, I felt awkward out there. I was big! What beach babe would look my way? The beach tempted me, but it took a pair of size 46 pants to actually change me. They were the largest size available in my school-issued baseball uniforms—and they were tight. I felt as if I'd hit a physical and emotional limit.

### HOW I CHANGED

My college was known for good food, which meant temptation was everywhere. So I set a few rules for myself: One, eat at least a palm-size portion of protein at every meal. Two, eat vegetables regularly—and even try a new one every now and then. Three, eat a piece of fruit whenever a snack craving hit. Amazingly, that's all it took for me to start losing weight.

A buddy joined me at the gym for my first cou-ple of trips, which was a great way to start out. He taught me some basic weight exercises, which made me feel less awkward. And when I hopped on the elliptical, I fell in love with a good sweat. The machine was easy on my knees, unlike running, and I could push myself to go 5 more minutes each time I exercised. Soon I moved to light jogging on the treadmill and then to running outdoors around campus. I was always increasing the challenge.

### THE REWARD

Freshman year I had a crush on a girl who wouldn't even look at me. By junior year, we were dating. We're no longer together, but the relationship was still a reward for my hard work. And with my new job as a personal trainer in New York City, I'm not lacking for Friday night dates. I tell my clients that I used to be big, and they can't imagine it. But when they eventually believe me, they start to believe in themselves, too.

## Palm Your Protein

The thickness and size of an average man's palm is about the size of 4 ounces of meat—or roughly 30 grams of protein, says Belly Off! nutritionist Christopher Mohr, PhD. Aim to include that size portion in every meal. If you do, Mohr says, you'll stay fuller for longer, which means you'll be less likely to give in to cravings.

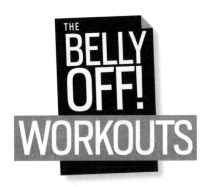

# Chapter 5

# THE BELLY OFF! INTERMEDIATE BACK-IN-SHAPE WORKOUT

A t least 6 weeks down and how many pounds lost? Congratulations! You have our permission to celebrate with your first beer or glass of wine in 6 weeks, if you are so inclined, or to have some other reward. If you are just coming off of the Beginner Back-in-Shape Workout, take 3 days to a full week off to recover before starting this intermediate workout.

During that time, keep up with your morning Beginner 2-Minute Drill. By now it should be as routine as brushing your teeth.

If you skipped the Beginner workout and are starting at the Intermediate level, we assume that you have been exercising regularly for more than 3 months and want to begin with something a little more challenging. If you aren't sure where to start, we recommend the Beginner program for everyone. But it's your choice.

Like the Beginner program, the Intermediate workout is also a metabolic-style program using mostly bodyweight strength exercises and calisthenics. But the Intermediate workout requires more from your body and brain than the Beginner workout does.

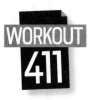

- Perform three different strength workouts each week, along with two cardio sessions. On strength workout days or rest days, do the walking program of your choice.

- Before each workout, warmup with the Intermediate 2-Minute Drill at 60 to 70 percent effort. You can perform some light cardio before the drill if you feel sore, tight, or tired.

- Perform the Belly Off! Intermediate Flex Series with the new booster moves described below, followed by the workout of the day.

- Important: As tempted as you'll be to dive right into the strength workout, do not skip these warmups, which will ready your body for work and protect you from injury.

- Cool down with another round of either the Flex Series or 3 minutes of walking. Your choice. Ideally, you should do both if you have the time.

# BELLY OFF! INTERMEDIATE FLEX SERIES

Perform the exercises on pages 90 and 91 as listed. Remember that doing these before your workouts will properly prepare you for your training and begin to positively affect your overall quality of life, as well. Try to fit them into your daily life. They will:

1. Help combat the traditional daily patterns that negatively affect posture and general health.

2. Increase nerve, joint, and muscle awareness.

3. Increase your heart rate and core temperature slowly and safely.

4. Transition the focus of your mind and body from the world around you to the task at hand—training properly. Exercising without warming up is an ineffective training model.

You'll find the descriptions of the Beginner Flex Series moves on page 63. Some of the moves designed for the Intermediate workout are more challenging variations on the Beginner flex moves, while others are new additions. You will use the Intermediate Flex Series in the Advanced workout, as well.

## GET JACKED!

### Greater Gains from Perfect Form

Be sure to take the time to learn the exercises and perform them properly. That's the key to safe, smart, effective training. As a trainer, I tell my clients that exercises work well when done properly. If your form is sloppy, you run the risk of injury, develop bad habits, and severely limit your progress. I've seen it happen again and again. The bigger crime is that you will spend your valuable time exercising for the sake of exercise, without intention and purpose. Get the patterns right, train them well, and your progress will skyrocket.

—David Jack

# WRIST ROLL
## FORWARD AND BACK, 10 REPS EACH WAY

See page 63 for directions.

# SHOULDER ROLL
## FORWARD AND BACK, 10 REPS EACH WAY

See page 63 for directions.

# ARM CIRCLE
## 15 REPS EACH WAY

Extend your arms out to your sides with your thumbs pointing forward. Keep your chest up, head in line with your body, and shoulders down (not shrugged) and make small, quick, but deliberate circles, trying to make even smaller circles with your hands. The movement comes from driving your thumbs forward or backward, depending on the direction of the circles, and being aware of your shoulders' role in the movement. Rotate your arms so your thumbs point behind you and repeat.

# HIP CIRCLE WITH BALANCE
## 10 REPS WITH EACH LEG

Follow the directions on page 63, but do 5 reps with your hands on a wall and 5 reps without support, balancing on one leg. Repeat with the other leg. Stay close to the wall in case you lose your balance.

# ANKLE CIRCLE
## 20 REPS WITH EACH FOOT

Follow the directions on page 64, but balance on one leg without the support of your hands on the wall.

# TWIST AND PRESS
## 10 REPS WITH EACH LEG FORWARD

Follow the directions on page 64, but instead of using a base stance, with your feet side by side, use a split stance, with one foot forward and one back. Focus on moving from your upper back, and try to avoid rotating your lower spine. (A slight rotation is okay, but not much.) Perform 15 reps with one leg forward, switch sides, and repeat.

# SINGLE LEG THREE-WAY STEP WITH HOP
## 5 REPS PER LEG

Follow the directions on page 64, but perform a small, controlled hop between each rep. Be sure to pause as you return your foot to center, dip at your hip and knee, and hop off the ground on one leg. Land softly on the ball of your foot first, with your following, so your full foot is on the ground as your hip and knee bend together to absorb the force.

# STANDING QUAD STRETCH
## 8 REPS PER LEG

Follow the directions on page 65, but perform the exercise without supporting yourself with your hands on a wall. Perform all reps with one leg, then repeat while balancing on the opposite leg.

# ISOMETRIC DOORWAY SPREAD APART
## 5 REPS WITH EACH ARM

Follow the directions on page 65, but use one arm at a time. Perform 5 reps with a 5-second hold with each arm. Use the leg opposite your working arm to drive into the floor and create support and power for the move. Avoid torquing or rotating your body.

# ISOMETRIC DOORWAY CHEST FLY
## 5 REPS WITH EACH ARM

Follow the directions on page 65, but use one arm at a time. Be sure to use the leg on the same side as your working arm for support, and drive your foot into the floor. Do not allow your body to torque or twist. Perform 5 reps with a 5-second hold, rest for 5 seconds, and repeat on the opposite side.

# THE 6-WEEK INTERMEDIATE STRENGTH WORKOUT

**Find Your Master Set:** Two or three days before your first workout, determine your "master set," the maximum number of repetitions you can do with good form for the following exercises in this order: Pushup, Inverted Row, Power Squat, and Alternating Reverse Lunge to Kick with your dominant leg forward. (When doing the Pushup and Inverted Row, pick an angle that allows you to do at least 8 reps.) Again, be sure to use a full range of motion and do as many as you can until you either feel you need to change your form in order to keep going or you need to rest. Do no more than a maximum of 20 pushups, 15 power squats and inverted rows, and 12 alternating reverse lunges. (Refer to pages 69, 70, 72, and 77 for more details on how to perform these exercises properly.)

## Weeks 1 to 6 Workout Schedule

| MONDAY | TUESDAY | WEDNESDAY | THURSDAY | FRIDAY | SATURDAY | SUNDAY |
|---|---|---|---|---|---|---|
| Strength Workout A | Cardio Workout: High-Intensity Interval (page 123) | Strength Workout B | Cardio Workout: Recovery Walk (page 124) | Strength Workout C | Cardio Workout: Steady State Aerobic (page 124) | Rest* or sports |

* Always rest for 1 day between strength workouts, but continue with daily walking.

# Strength Workout A

This will be your first workout of the week every week for the next 6 weeks. Workout A is designed to prepare your body for Workouts B and C. It employs exercises that move your body dynamically in various planes of motion to boost heart rate and metabolism and tap into fast-twitch muscle fibers (the ones responsible for quick, explosive bursts of power) to drive muscle growth and improve the strength of your connective tissue.

# WEEKS 1 AND 2

# WORKOUT A
## WARMUP
Intermediate 2-Minute Drill (see page 40)
Intermediate Flex Series (see page 89)

| STRENGTH PREP | REPS | SETS |
|---|---|---|
| REVERSE LUNGE TO KICK | 5 (each leg) | 1 |
| POWER SQUAT JUMP | 5 | 3 (30 sec. rest in between) |
| LATERAL SKATE BOUND | 8 (each direction) | |
| STRENGTH EXERCISES | REPS | ROUNDS |
| BLOCK 1 | | As many as possible in 3 minutes |
| INVERTED ROW | Master set | |
| POWER SQUAT | Master set | |
| SPLIT JACK | 16 | |
| BLOCK 2 | | As many as possible in 3 minutes |
| PUSHUP | Master set | |
| ALTERNATING REVERSE LUNGE AND HOLD | Master set | |
| SKIP IN PLACE | 30 | |
| BLOCK 3 | Repeat Block 1 exercises | |
| BLOCK 4 | Repeat Block 2 exercises | |

# COOLDOWN
Walk (3 minutes)
Intermediate Flex Series (see page 89)

**WORKOUT A PROGRESSIONS: WEEKS 3 TO 6**
Increase each strength exercise by 2 reps every week.

STRENGTH PREP

# REVERSE LUNGE TO KICK

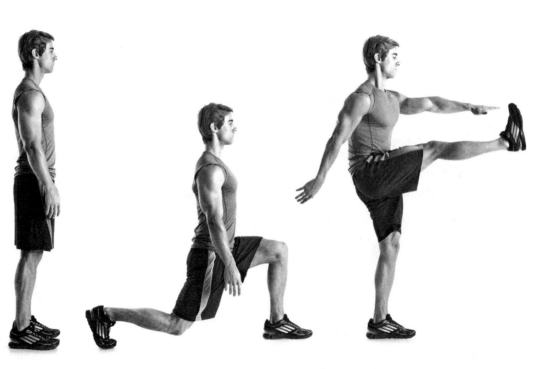

Stand with your legs shoulder-width apart. Take a step backward with your right foot and lower yourself into a lunge position—your right knee should almost touch the ground and your left thigh should be parallel to the ground. Keep your back straight and make sure your left knee doesn't extend past your toes. You will feel tension in your left thigh and calf and glutes. Keep your left foot flat on the ground. Immediately swing your right leg forward, standing up as fast as possible while maintaining a strong, steady body line. Swing your right leg straight out in front of you until your opposite hand touches your swinging leg. Do the 5 reps quickly, then step back with your left foot and repeat the swing and touch with your left leg and right arm.

## STRENGTH PREP

# POWER SQUAT JUMP

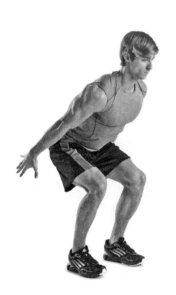
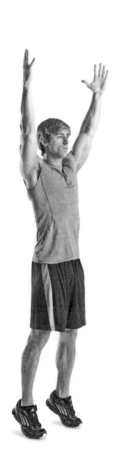
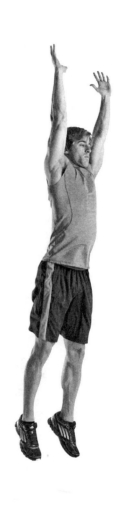

Stand with your feet slightly more than shoulder-width apart, toes forward, hands outstretched above your head. Simultaneously push your hips back and swing your arms down to your sides, pulling your body down until your thighs are nearly parallel to the floor. Immediately drive your hands up toward the sky as you extend your body and jump off the ground. As you land, the balls of your feet should touch first followed by your heels. Pull your arms down and sit back again. Repeat 4 more times. Rest. Repeat for 5 reps. Rest. Repeat for 5 reps. Throughout the movement, be sure to keep your chest up and knees over your ankles, and use your arms forcefully.

### STRENGTH PREP

# LATERAL SKATER BOUND

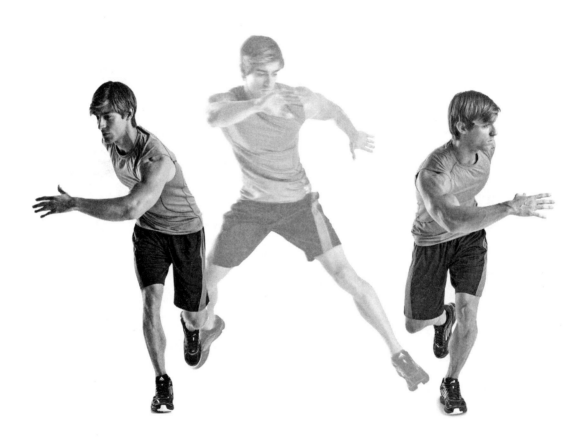

Stand with your feet hip-width apart, knees and arms slightly bent, leaning forward a bit at your waist. Leap laterally to the right at least 2 feet and allow your left foot to swing behind you and outside your right foot. Immediately bound back to your left, landing on your left foot and allowing your right foot to swing behind your left leg. The exercise is similar to a speed skater's side-to-side movement, and as such should involve swinging your arms for momentum. Be sure to push the ground away from you with your outside leg and land by bending your hip and knee. Continue back and forth this way for 8 large bounds on each side.

# How to Do the Strength Blocks

## BLOCK 1

Perform the following exercises in order, completing the required reps before moving to the next exercise. Rest between exercises as needed. Do as many rounds of Block 1 as you can in 3 minutes.

- Inverted Row, master set (see page 77)
- Power Squat, master set (see page 70)
- Split Jack, 16 reps

After 3 minutes, stop and rest for 2 minutes. While resting, chart the number of rounds you completed. Note how you felt. With each subsequent week's Workout A, try to do "more work," that is, more Block 1 rounds without sacrificing form. Charting or journaling your workouts is a good way to track your personal records.

## BLOCK 2

Perform the following exercises in order, completing the required reps before moving to the next exercise. Rest between exercises as needed. Do as many rounds of Block 2 as you can in 3 minutes.

- Pushup, master set (see page 72)
- Alternating Reverse Lunge, master set (see page 69)
- Skip in Place, 30 reps (each step equals 1 rep)

After 3 minutes, stop and rest for 2 minutes. While resting, chart the number of rounds you completed. Note how you felt. With each subsequent week's Workout A, try to do "more work," that is, more Block 2 rounds without sacrificing form. Chart the number of rounds completed.

## BLOCK 3

Repeat Block 1 exercises (Inverted Row, Power Squat, Split Jack).

## BLOCK 4

Repeat Block 2 exercises (Pushup, Alternating Reverse Lunge, Skip in Place).

**HEALTH**
Work Out
Your
Demons

Regular aerobic exercise can be as effective as taking antidepressant medication, according to a study at the University of Texas Southwestern Medical Center.

## BLOCK 1

# SPLIT JACK

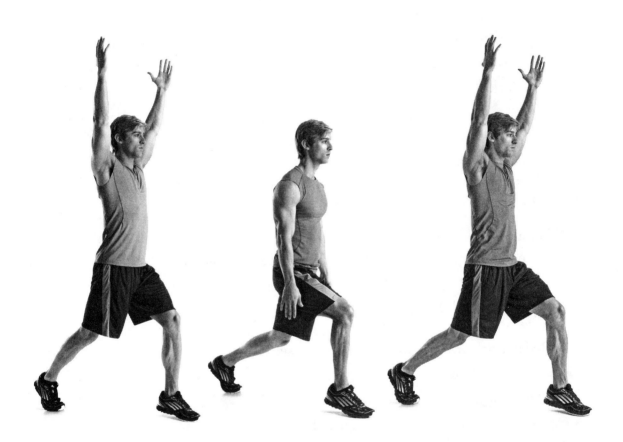

Stand with your feet hip-width apart and your arms at your sides as you would to begin a jumping jack. Instead of jumping and splitting your legs to the sides, make a small jump to split your legs—left leg forward, right leg back while swinging your arms out and overhead as in a traditional jumping jack. Land on the balls of both feet, knees slightly bent. Immediately swing your arms down to your sides as you jump and switch leg positions—right leg forward, left leg back. That's 1 rep. Continue to alternate feet with each jump as you swing your arms up and down to your sides.

# THE 6-WEEK PROGRESSION

Increase each block training time as follows in Weeks 2 through 6:

**Week 2:** 4 minutes

**Week 3:** 5 minutes

**Week 4:** 2 rounds, 3 minutes each; rest 90 seconds between rounds

**Week 5:** 2 rounds, 4 minutes each; rest 90 seconds between rounds

**Week 6:** 3 rounds, 2 minutes each round, resting 60 seconds between rounds

**FIT FACT**

# 1,095

Estimated number of days you can add to your life by exercising for just 15 minutes a day over a 13-year period, according to a study in the medical journal the *Lancet*. Exercise reduces risk of heart disease, diabetes, and cancer.

# Strength Workout B

This workout includes a series of core exercises, two metabolic strength circuits, and a challenging finisher, just for pure, sweat-inducing fun!

## WEEKS 1 TO 2

## WORKOUT B

### WARMUP

Intermediate 2-Minute Drill (see page 40) + Intermediate Flex Series (see page 89)

| CORE EXERCISES* | REPS/TIME | SETS |
|---|---|---|
| PLANK | 30 seconds | 1 |
| GLUTE BRIDGE | 8 reps | 1 |
| SIDE PLANK (RIGHT) | 20 seconds | 1 |
| SUPERMAN | 8 reps | 1 |
| SIDE PLANK (LEFT) | 20 seconds | 1 |
| STRENGTH EXERCISES** | REPS | ROUNDS |
| CIRCUIT 1 | | |
| REVERSE PUSHUP | As many as possible in 30 seconds | 2 |
| SPLIT STANCE ISOMETRIC TOWEL ROW | 5 reps each leg | 2 |
| REVERSE LUNGE WITH KNEE DRIVE | 15 seconds each leg | 2 |
| CIRCUIT 2 | | |
| LATERAL LUNGE | 15 seconds each leg | 2 |
| KNEELING CHOP | 15 seconds to each side | 2 |
| SHOULDER ELEVATED HIP THRUST | As many as possible in 30 seconds | 2 |
| FINISHER | | |
| TOWEL WAVE | 100 | 1 |

* Rest 15 seconds between exercises. Discontinue workout if experiencing low-back pain.
**Rest 45 seconds between exercises; 90–120 seconds between rounds.

### COOLDOWN

Walk (3 minutes) + Intermediate Flex Series (see page 89)
See Weeks 3 to 6 Progression (see page 105)

## CORE EXERCISE

# PLANK

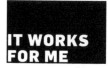

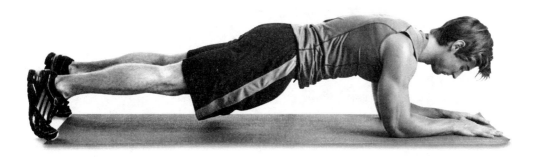

Start to get into a pushup position, but bend your elbows and rest your weight on your forearms, instead of your hands. Your body should form a straight line from your shoulders to your ankles. Brace your core by contracting your abs as if you were about to be punched in the gut and squeeze your glutes and thighs. Hold this position for 30 seconds while taking short powerful breaths.

## CORE EXERCISE

# GLUTE BRIDGE

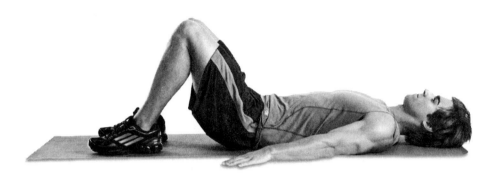

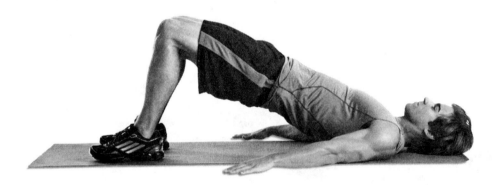

Lie on your back with your knees bent and your arms and heels on the floor. Press your hands, palms down, into the floor hard. At the same time, push down through your heels and squeeze your glutes to raise your body into a straight line from knees to shoulders. Pause at the top for 2 seconds before lowering and repeating. Avoid arching your lower back. Do 8 reps.

## CORE EXERCISE

# SIDE PLANK

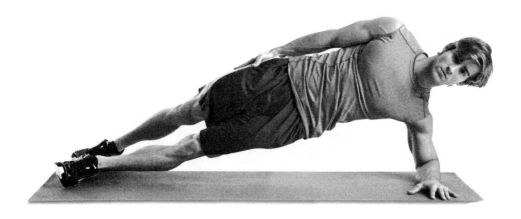

Lie on your left side with your legs straight, your right leg on top of your left. Prop your upper body up on your left elbow and forearm. Position your elbow under your shoulder. Brace your core by contracting your abs forcefully. Raise your hips until your body forms a straight line from your ankles to your shoulders. Your head should stay in line with your body. Hold this position for 20 seconds while taking short powerful breaths. Repeat the side plank hold on your right side.

## CORE EXERCISE

# SUPERMAN

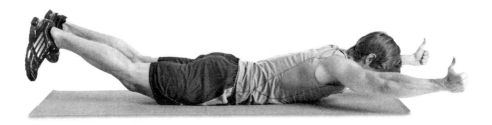

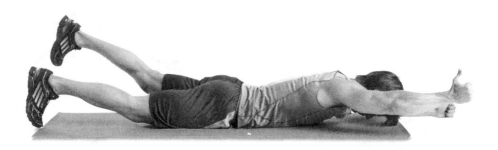

Lie facedown with your arms extended straight overhead, your legs extended straight. Simultaneously lift your head, chest, arms, and legs up, so you're in a Supermanlike flying position. Hold this position for 2 seconds, then relax your arms and legs to the floor and repeat. *Note:* If this Superman move is difficult, try the Alternating Diagonal Superman (see second photograph above), where you leave one arm and the opposite leg on the floor and raise only the opposing arm and leg. Hold the lift, relax down to the floor, and lift your other arm and leg. Squeeze glutes to protect the low back. Do 8 reps.

# Strength Circuits

Perform each exercise in Circuit 1 as many times as you can in 30 seconds, then rest for 45 seconds before starting the next exercise. Rest for 90 to 120 seconds, and then repeat Circuit 1.

Next, move to Circuit 2, following the same pattern as 1, resting 45 seconds between exercises and 90 to 120 seconds between circuits. Note: With each subsequent week, you will adjust the exercise or rest times. See the 6-Week Progression, below.

## CIRCUIT 1

- Reverse Pushup
- Split Stance Isometric Towel Row
- Reverse Lunge with Knee Drive

## CIRCUIT 2

- Lateral Lunge
- Kneeling Chop
- Shoulder Elevated Hip Thrust

# WEEKS 3 TO 6 PROGRESSIONS

**Week 3:** 40 seconds on, 60 seconds off—2 rounds of each circuit

**Week 4:** 50 seconds on, 50 seconds off—2 rounds of each circuit

**Week 5:** 30 seconds on, 30 seconds off—3 rounds of each circuit

**Week 6:** 50 seconds on, 60 seconds off—3 rounds of each circuit

### CIRCUIT 1

## REVERSE PUSHUP

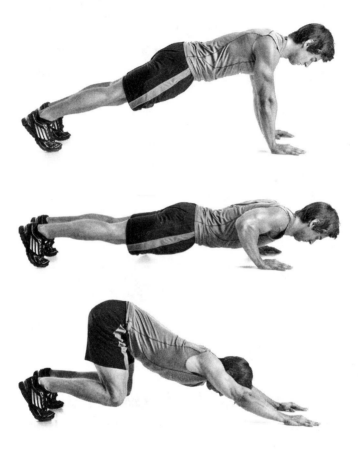

Assume a pushup position, with your hands directly under your shoulders and your toes anchored to the floor behind you. Your body should be straight from head to heels. Now lower your body with control. Here's where it gets different: Instead of pushing yourself up, as you would for a standard pushup, bend your knees and push your body backward, almost scraping the floor with your nose. (This move mimics an overhead shoulder press, but your hands are on the floor.) Then, dig your toes into the floor and explosively straighten your legs to push yourself back into the top pushup position. Lock your shoulders so your momentum doesn't drive them beyond directly above your hands. Pause, then repeat. Once you get accustomed to the movement, do it quickly.

**CIRCUIT 1**

# SPLIT STANCE ISOMETRIC TOWEL ROW

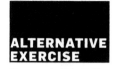

**ALTERNATIVE EXERCISE**

You can do this Split Stance Isometric Row with dumbbells. Do 10 reps and pause at the top for 3 seconds.

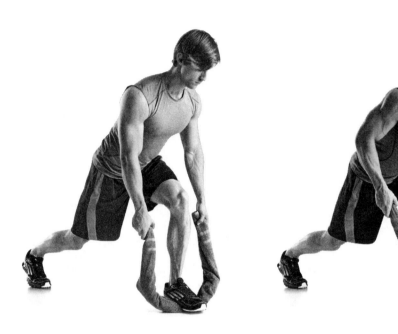

Using both hands, grab a 4-foot length of rope or a bath towel rolled up into a rope shape. Assume a split stance with your left foot forward. Slip the middle of the rope or towel under your front foot to anchor it. Lean forward slightly, choke up your grip on the towel or rope, and pull the ends of the rope or towel toward your ribs. Open your chest and pull your elbows back away from your foot as you would during a bent-over row. This is an isometric exercise. Pull as hard as you can while pressing your foot into the rope or towel to secure it in place. Hold for 3 seconds, and then release. Do 10 reps of 3-second holds, switching legs after 5 reps and anchoring the rope or towel with your right foot forward.

## CIRCUIT 1

# REVERSE LUNGE WITH KNEE DRIVE

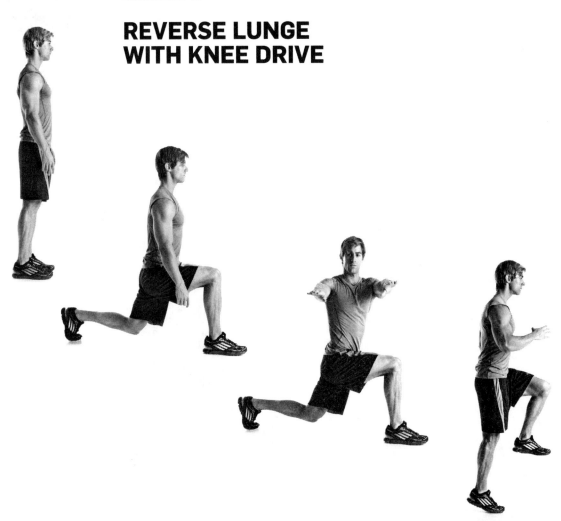

Perform a reverse lunge by stepping back with your left leg and lowering until your back knee nearly touches the floor and your right knee is bent at 90 degrees. Extend your arms in front of you and parallel to the floor. Then rotate your arms and torso right across your lead leg. Return to center and push explosively through both legs until you are standing (still in the split stance). When your legs are straight, lift your back (left) knee and drive it forward and up to your chest, then immediately lower it back to the rear lunge position. Repeat this sequence quickly for 15 seconds and then switch leg positions and perform the move with your left leg forward.

## CIRCUIT 2

# LATERAL LUNGE

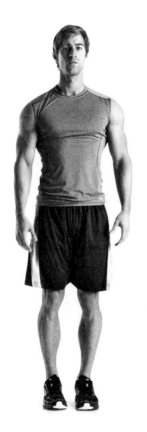

Stand with your feet hip-width apart and your hands at your sides. Keeping your toes pointed forward, take an exaggerated step to your right and sit down and back on your right leg, keeping your chest up and left leg straight. Extend your arms in front of you for balance. Pause for 2 seconds, then press your right foot into the floor to push yourself back to the starting position and repeat. Do repetitions to the right for 15 seconds, then to the left for 15 seconds, remembering to pause for 2 seconds while you're in the lunge.

**CIRCUIT 2**

# KNEELING CHOP

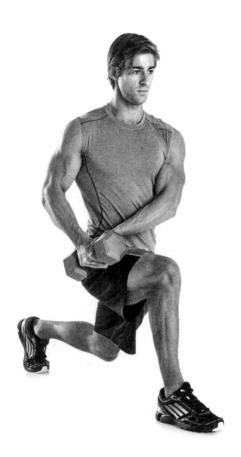

Grasp a dumbbell with both hands, and raise the dumbbell above your left shoulder. Step forward with your right leg and kneel on your left knee. This is the starting position. Brace your core and squeeze your glutes. Now swing the dumbbell down and past your right hip without rotating your torso. Keep your torso upright and your arms mostly straight for the entire movement. Don't round your back. Return the weight to your left shoulder and repeat for 15 seconds. Then raise the weight over your right shoulder and kneel on your right knee and chop the dumbbell from your right shoulder past your left hip for 15 seconds.

**CIRCUIT 2**

# SHOULDER ELEVATED HIP THRUST

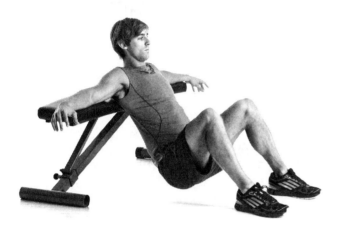

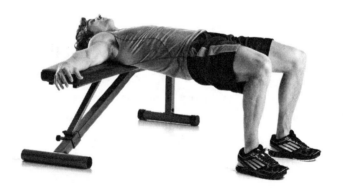

A cousin of the Glute Bridge, this move creates increased load and a greater range of hip motion. Sit on the floor with your back and shoulders up against an exercise bench or stationary chair or ottoman. Your legs should be bent, feet flat on the floor, chest out. Keeping your head in line with your torso, press your feet into the floor, squeeze your glutes, and push your hips toward the ceiling. The back of your shoulders will press into the bench or chair to support you. Stop when your chest, hips, and thighs are in a straight line. Do not arch your back. Pause here for a second, then slowly lower yourself until your butt touches the floor. Repeat fo 30 seconds. For greater resistance, you can hold a weight plate or sandbag on your chest.

## THE FINISHER

A "finisher" is a fast-paced metabolic ender for your workout that really boosts fat burn. We like to use battling ropes for finishers. These are long, thick, heavy-duty tug-of-war–style ropes that you swing up and down and side to side. Most boot camp gyms have them. If you don't have heavy-duty ropes at home, don't buy them. We have an easy way to mimic the battle rope burn: the Towel Wave!

## TOWEL WAVE

Grab the largest, thickest beach towel you can find. Hold the corners of one short end in each hand. (You'll find that rolling the corners up a bit in each hand will improve your grip.) Standing with your feet shoulder-width apart and knees slightly bent, lift and drop your hands to make waves with the towel as if you're shaking sand out of it. Find a rhythm to make a fluid wave. Avoid shrugging your shoulders and leaning too far forward or backward. Relax your head and neck as much as possible. The towel wave may seem easy at first, but you'll be huffing and puffing at the end. Do 100 towel waves as quickly as possible. Rest if you need to. Every week, increase the number of waves by 10 reps.

# Intermediate Workout C

Welcome to the Trifecta, in which we combine three different training styles within a circuit to shock your system into greater muscle growth. The Trifecta circuits include isometric holds, bodyweight strength patterns, and locomotion exercises to ignite fat burn. The workout progresses over the course of the 6 weeks to ensure that you do more—and harder—work as time passes.

## THE TRIFECTA CIRCUITS

There are 3 different circuits described here. Perform 2 rounds of each circuit as quickly as possible, resting up to 30 seconds between each exercise. Rest for 90 seconds between rounds. After completing 2 rounds of Circuit 1, rest for 90 seconds, and move to Circuit 2, and so on. Chart how long it takes you to complete both rounds of each circuit. For the Split Squat Isometric Holds in Circuit 1, switch your forward leg on the second round.

# WEEK 1
# WORKOUT C
## WARMUP
Intermediate 2-Minute Drill (see page 40)
Intermediate Flex Series (see page 89)

| STRENGTH EXERCISES * | REPS/TIME | ROUNDS |
|---|---|---|
| **TRIFECTA CIRCUIT 1** | | 2 |
| **DOWN DOG PUSHUP** | 10 reps | |
| **SPLIT SQUAT ISOMETRIC HOLD** | 30 seconds each leg | |
| **QUICK FEET** | 10 reps with each leg leading | |
| **TRIFECTA CIRCUIT 2** | | 2 |
| **SPLIT STANCE BAND ROW** | 10 each side | |
| **ISOMETRIC PUSHUP HOLD** | 30 seconds | |
| **THREE-WAY JUMP** | 10 reps | |
| **TRIFECTA CIRCUIT 3** | | 2 |
| **EXPLOSIVE STEPUP JUMP** | 10 reps each leg | |
| **ISOMETRIC SUMO SQUAT** | 30 seconds | |
| **MULE KICK** | 10 reps | |

*Rest 30 seconds between exercises; rest 90 seconds between rounds.

# COOLDOWN
Walk (3 minutes)
Intermediate Flex Series (see page 89)

### WORKOUT C PROGRESSIONS: WEEKS 2 TO 6

**Weeks 2 and 3:** Add 1 rep to each exercise per week; increase length of isometric holds by 10 to 30 seconds.

**Week 4:** Add a third round to each circuit, but reduce the reps and time per exercise to the level of Week 1.

**Weeks 5 and 6:** Add 1 rep to each exercise per week; increase the length of the isometric holds by 10 seconds per week. Do 3 rounds of each circuit.

### CIRCUIT 1

# DOWN DOG PUSHUP

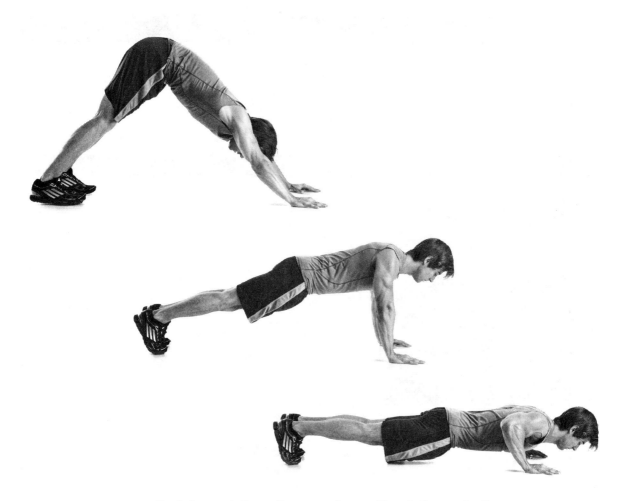

Begin in yoga's Down Dog pose, feet and hands flat on the floor, arms and legs straight, hips lifted up toward the ceiling, spine straight, and head in line with your back. Your feet are slightly wider than hip-width apart. (If you need to lift your heels slightly off the floor or bend your knees, that's okay.) This is the starting position. Now, lower your hips under control until you are in the standard pushup position. Do a full pushup, and then, from the top pushup position, dip your head through your hands as you lift your hips back into the Down Dog position again. Repeat. Do 10 reps.

**CIRCUIT 1**

# SPLIT SQUAT ISOMETRIC HOLD

## WEIGHT LOSS

## The Shut-Eye Workout

If you've been burning the midnight oil, you'd be better off sleeping than getting up early for a workout. Sleep deprivation can derail your weight-loss efforts by slowing metabolism and increasing appetite, according to researchers at the University of Chicago.

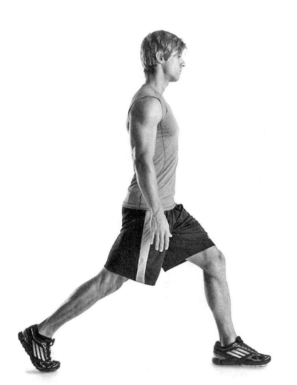

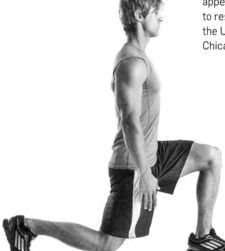

Assume a split squat with your left foot forward and flat on the ground and your right foot about 3 feet behind it. Lower into a squat until your front leg is bent at 90 degrees and your back knee is hovering just above the floor. Hold this position for 30 seconds. Stand up and shake your legs out if needed. Then switch your foot positions, bringing your right foot forward this time. Squat and hold for 30 seconds.

## CIRCUIT 1

# QUICK FEET

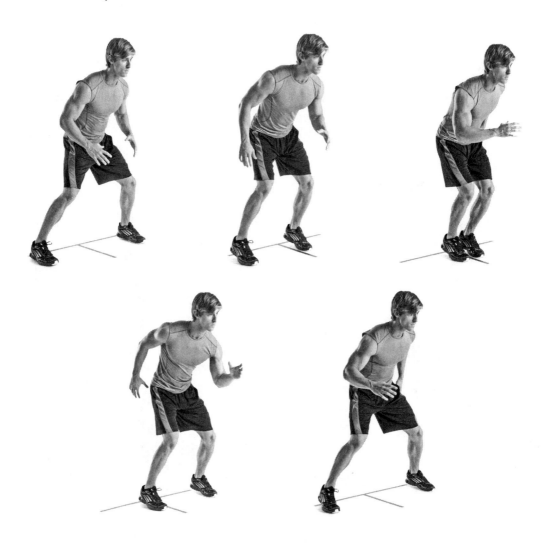

Stand with your feet at least shoulder-width apart, knees slightly bent, hips back a bit, and chest up. Imagine a line between your feet. Now, using a four-step count, quickly step your left foot in toward the line, then your right, then step out with your left foot, then step your right foot out. That's 1 rep. Perform 10 reps, rest briefly, and repeat, leading with your right foot.

**CIRCUIT 2**

# SPLIT STANCE BAND ROW

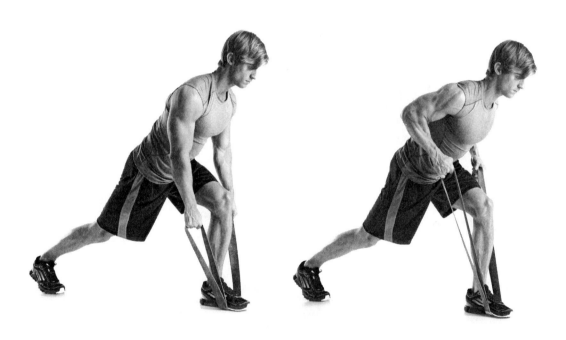

Split your stance so your left foot is forward and standing on the middle of an exercise band and your right foot is about 3 feet behind you. Lean forward and rise up onto the ball of your back foot. Grasp each end of the exercise band in your right hand. Pull the band to the sides of your rib cage, keeping your elbows in close to your body. Pull until your bent elbows reach just past your back, and then allow the band to pull your hands back to the starting position, and repeat. Do 10 reps. Switch foot positions to step on the band with your right foot and repeat the exercise.

## CIRCUIT 2

# ISOMETRIC PUSHUP HOLD

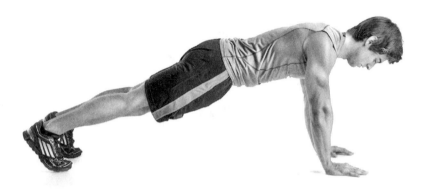

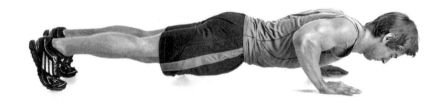

Assume the top pushup position with arms straight. Lower yourself into the down position, your nose hovering just above the floor and your elbows tucked against your sides. Squeeze your glutes and shoulder blades together and draw your belly button toward your spine. Hold this position for 30 seconds. Rest as needed but only count time toward your 30 seconds when in the hold.

**CIRCUIT 2**

# THREE-WAY JUMP

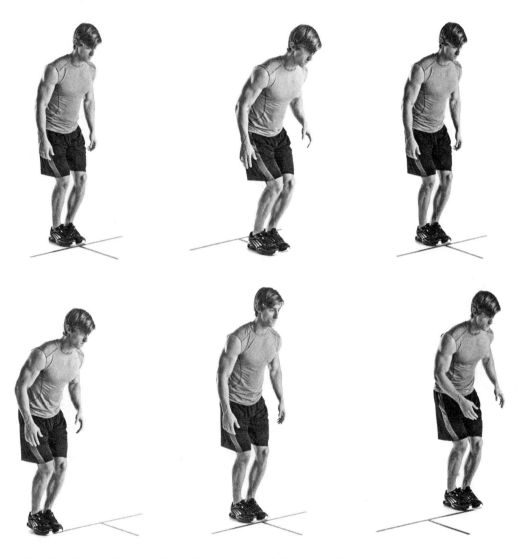

Stand with your feet together. Using small, quick hops and keeping your feet together, jump forward and then immediately jump back. Then jump about a foot to your right and then back to center. Jump left and back to center. That's 1 rep. Then jump backward, then left, then right. Keep alternating this way for 10 reps.

## CIRCUIT 3

# EXPLOSIVE STEPUP JUMP

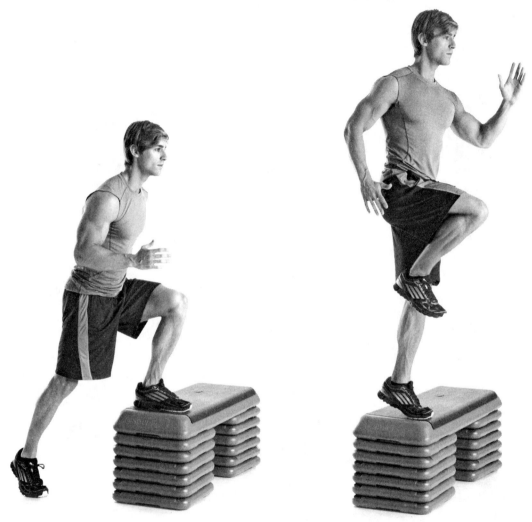

Stand with your left foot on an exercise bench or step that's about 18 inches high. Press into the step with your foot to raise your body. As your left leg straightens, drive your right knee up until your thigh is parallel to the floor. Lower your right foot to the floor without taking your left off the bench. Do 10 repetitions quickly. Switch foot positions and do 10 reps on the opposite side.

**CIRCUIT 3**

# ISOMETRIC SUMO SQUAT

**FIT FACT**
# 8.5
Percentage increase in your metabolism if you eat 18 grams of protein prior to a training session, according to the journal *Medicine and Science in Sports and Exercise*.

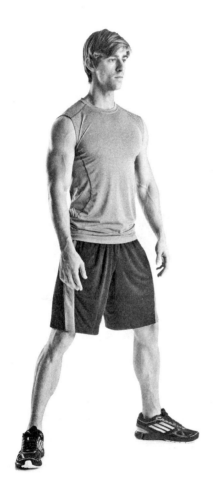
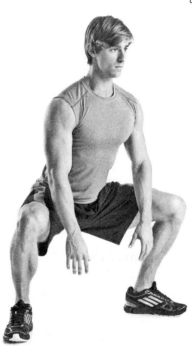

Stand with your feet about twice shoulder-width apart, your toes turned out. Lower your body by pushing your hips back and bending your knees. Keep your abs tight and torso upright with your lower back naturally arched. The tops of your thighs should be parallel with the floor or lower with your feet flat on the floor and knees outward. Hold this position for 30 seconds, then push yourself up to the starting position.

## CIRCUIT 3

# MULE KICK

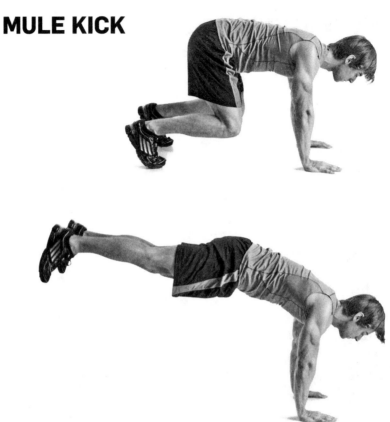

Start in a bear crawl position, with your knees bent at 90 degrees (but not touching the floor) and your hands on the floor under your shoulders. Now contract your core and glutes and kick both feet up and back into the air, straightening your legs and quickly bending them again so that you land softly on the balls of your feet. That's 1 rep. Do 10 reps. If this move is too difficult, try kicking one leg back at a time (below), leaving the opposite leg in the bent position. Alternate legs.

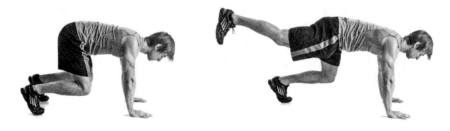

# INTERMEDIATE CARDIO WORKOUTS

In the intermediate program, you'll do three different cardio workouts per week—a high-intensity interval, a steady-state aerobic, and a light recovery walk workout. Do them on the days when you aren't doing a resistance-training workout. Warm up with a Belly Off! 2-Minute Drill before each cardio session.

## HIGH-INTENSITY INTERVAL

This is the cardio workout in which you will push yourself the hardest. We use an interval style called a fartlek, which is Swedish for "speed play." These workouts are short, lasting just 20 to 25 minutes. We'll describe a running fartlek here, but you can also do fartleks on a bicycle or a piece of cardio equipment, or even by mixing walking with running.

Start with 5 minutes of slow jogging to warm up. Increase your speed to a moderate level for about 1 minute. Then run hard at a level of 7 or 8, on a scale where 10 is an all-out sprint. When you tire, slow down to an exertion level of 3 or 4 to recover. Your bouts of intense running may be 30 seconds to a minute long, but don't worry about timing yourself. Just follow how your body feels. Slow down when you feel the need to and take as much time as you need to recover and be ready for intense effort again. Otherwise you will end up blending the speeds together and turning the workout into a steady-state run. Use the last 3 to 5 minutes of your workout to slowly cool down.

Here is your 6-week plan for your interval cardio days:

**Week 1:** 20 minutes          **Week 4:** 20 minutes
**Week 2:** 20 minutes          **Week 5:** 25 minutes
**Week 3:** 25 minutes          **Week 6:** 20 minutes

Chart your distance each workout and seek to beat it during subsequent workouts. A great goal is to travel as far in Week 6 in 20 minutes as you did in Week 3 in 25 minutes.

## STEADY-STATE AEROBIC

For this workout, choose a trail or route or type of cardio equipment that's different from where you went or what you did on your Interval Day. Start with a 5-minute slow warmup, then increase your effort level to a 6 or 7 on an exertion scale of 1 to 10, where 10 is a sprint. At 6 or 7, you should be able to speak in a few short sentences but it shouldn't be comfortable to talk for long. Progress as follows through the 6 weeks.

**Week 1:** 20 minutes

**Week 2:** 22 minutes

**Week 3:** 24 minutes

**Week 4:** 26 minutes

**Week 5:** 28 minutes

**Week 6:** 30 minutes

## RECOVERY WALK

Do a brisk 20- to 30-minute walk with a friend (four-legged or two).

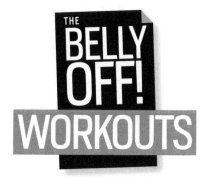

# Chapter 6

# THE BELLY OFF! ADVANCED BACK-IN-SHAPE WORKOUT

The investment banker in you may want to start your plan to get back in shape with the Advanced workout. We applaud your warrior instinct, but before you leapfrog over the Beginner and Intermediate programs, we encourage you to make sure the following things are true:

- You have been training consistently 3 or more days each week for at least 3 months.
- You possess a solid base of bodyweight strength and pain-free movement.
- You have good aerobic endurance.
- You have good mobility in your ankle, knee, hip, and shoulder joints.
- You haven't been ill or injured recently.

If you can't meet all five of these criteria, take a step back to at least the Intermediate workout and save yourself some pain.

But if you have completed the Beginner and Intermediate workouts in this book, then you're ready. Listen to your body, and go at your own pace. That's the key to good training. The principles never change, though the methods and intensity might. It's time to buckle down on your diet and lifestyle changes, crank up these workouts for the next 6 weeks, and blast through plateaus.

- Perform 3 different strength-training workouts per week on nonconsecutive days.
- Do two 20- to 25-minute interval cardio sessions per week (choose running or cycling).
- Do one steady-state aerobic workout of 30 minutes every other week (such as moderate-pace running), taking a rest day on the off weeks.
- On the 7th day of training, go for a 60-minute power walk with a partner or play a sport with family or friends (tennis, basketball, racquetball, volleyball, touch football, baseball, etc.).
- Before each workout, warmup with the Advanced 2-Minute Drill at 60 to 70 percent of your maximum effort and the Belly Off! Intermediate Flex Series.

- Cool down with another round of the Advanced 2-Minute Drill and Flex Series.

# THE 6-WEEK ADVANCED STRENGTH WORKOUT

The advanced back-in-shape workout is a 6-week program made up of three different metabolic strength sessions—Workouts A, B, and C. You'll be active every single day of the week. The resistance training sessions are quick and tough. If you skip meals, don't get enough sleep, or don't drink enough water, you won't have the strength to get through this program. It's time to get after it!

## Weeks 1 to 6 Workout Schedule

| MONDAY | TUESDAY | WEDNESDAY | THURSDAY | FRIDAY | SATURDAY | SUNDAY |
|---|---|---|---|---|---|---|
| Strength Workout A | Cardio Workout: Interval Day 1 | Strength Workout B | Cardio Workout: Steady-State Aerobic | Strength Workout C | Cardio Workout: Interval Day 2 | Fun Fitness Day |

## STRENGTH PREP

Get your muscles ready for work with these two exercises: the Medicine Ball Scoop Toss and the Lateral Single-Leg Jump to Double Return. Do 3 sets of 10 repetitions of the medicine ball toss, followed by 2 sets of the lateral jumps. Rest for 30 seconds between sets.

## STRENGTH PREP

# MEDICINE BALL SCOOP TOSS

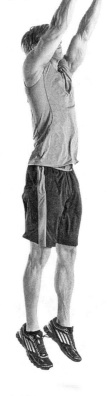

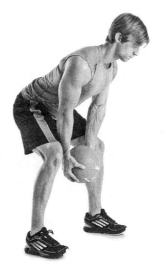

Stand in an open space holding a light medicine ball (4 to 8 pounds) in front of your body. Bend your knees slightly and push your hips back, keeping your chest up and back flat. Straighten your arms to lower the ball and, using a scooping motion while keeping your arms straight, throw the ball up as high as you can. Allow the ball to bounce on the ground one time, and then grab it with both hands. Set your feet and repeat the throw. Be sure to engage your core to stabilize your body as you throw. The power of the toss should come from your hips by driving your feet through the ground and driving your head up toward the sky. Do 10. You will also feel the throw from your upper back, and a bit in your lower, as well. You should not, however, feel pain in your lower back. *Note:* If you're doing this move in a room with a low ceiling, stand 6 to 8 feet away from a wall and bounce the medicine ball off of the wall.

**STRENGTH PREP**

# LATERAL SINGLE-LEG JUMP TO DOUBLE RETURN

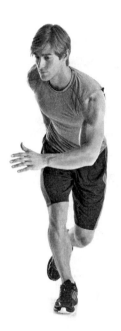 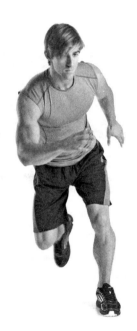 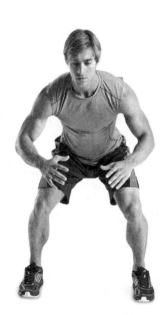

Stand with your feet hip-width apart, knees slightly bent, and torso bent forward a bit. Lift your left leg behind you and balance on your right. This is the starting position. Now powerfully drive your right foot into the ground to jump to your left. Land on your left foot, absorbing the impact by bending at your hip and knee, and quickly push off your left foot to jump back to the right, landing on both feet hip-width apart. (It's a single-leg takeoff and return, followed by a double-footed landing.) That's 1 rep. Perform 6, switch sides, and repeat. Rest for 60 seconds and repeat for a second set. Recover for 2 minutes before beginning the strength-training workout.

# Strength Workout A

There is a 2-move strength prep, 2 exercise blocks, and a challenge circuit in this workout. Do 1 set of the first exercise, then move to the next exercises and repeat. Rest for 45 seconds between exercises and 90 seconds between rounds.

## WEEKS 1 TO 3

### WARMUP

Advanced 2-Minute Drill (see page 49) + Intermediate Flex Series (see page 89)

| STRENGTH PREP | REPS | ROUNDS |
|---|---|---|
| MEDICINE BALL SCOOP TOSS | 10 | 3 |
| LATERAL SINGLE-LEG JUMP | 6 each direction | 2 |
| **STRENGTH EXERCISES** | **REPS** | **ROUNDS** |
| BLOCK 1 | | |
| ISO EXPLOSIVE SPLIT SQUAT | 21 | 2 |
| ISO STANDING BAND PRESS | 5 reps each arm | 2 |
| BLOCK 2 | | |
| SANDBAG ZERCHER SQUAT | 12 | 2 |
| NEIDLER PRESS WITH PLATE | 8 reps each side | 2 |
| BODYSAW | 10 | 2 |
| 2-MINUTE DRILL CHALLENGE | | 2 |
| JUMPING JACK | 10 | |
| PRISONER SQUAT | 10 | |
| HIGH-KNEE SKIP | 10 | |
| SIDE-TO-SIDE HOP | 10 | |
| PUSHUP | 10 | |
| CRUNCH | 10 | |
| MOUNTAIN CIMBER | 10 | |
| BODYWEIGHT THRUSTER | 10 | |

### COOLDOWN

Walk (3 minutes) + Intermediate Flex Series (see page 89)

**WORKOUT A PROGRESSIONS: WEEKS 4 TO 6**

Do 3 rounds of Blocks 1 and 2.

**BLOCK 1**

# ISOMETRIC EXPLOSIVE SPLIT SQUAT WITH MEDICINE BALL

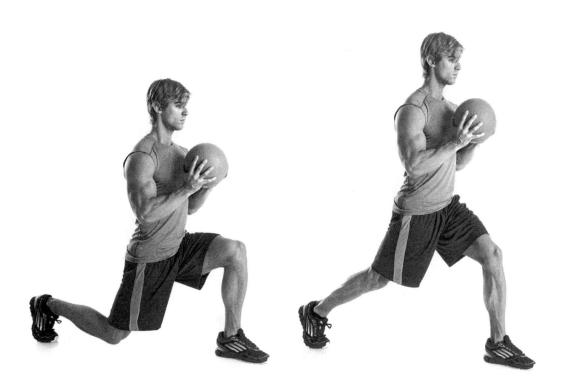

Get into a split squat position, with your left foot forward and flat on the ground and your shin almost perpendicular to the floor. Your back (right) knee hovers just above the floor. Keep your chest up and abs engaged. Hold this position for 6 seconds, then quickly straighten both legs and return to the split squat stance. Next, hold the bottom position for 5 seconds and perform 2 reps of the up and down split squat. Keep subtracting 1 second from your hold and adding 1 rep to your squats in this way so that your last hold is 1 second long, followed by 6 quick up-and-down reps. Choose a medicine ball or dumbbell weight that's heavy enough so that the last hold and reps are challenging but manageable to complete with good form. You will perform 21 total seconds of iso holds on each leg and 21 total reps of traditional up-and-down split squats. (To make this exercise is more difficult, hold the medicine ball with your arms extended straight in the up position.)

## BLOCK 1

# ISOMETRIC EXPLOSIVE STANDING BAND PRESS

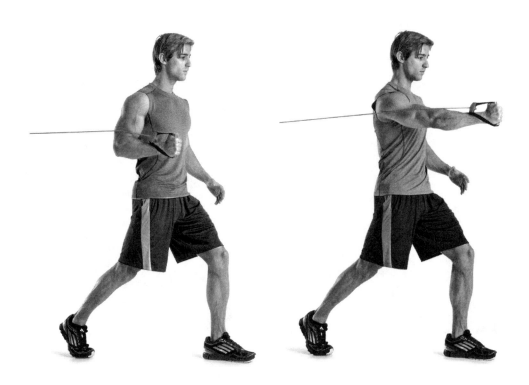

Secure the end of an exercise band to a stationary object, face away from the anchor point, and hold the band's handle in your right hand so the band is under tension and tucked up near your armpit. (Alternatively, you can use a cable station instead of a band.) Assume a split stance, with your left foot forward and your right foot back. This is the starting position. Press the band or cable forward until your arm is straight. Hold this position for a count of 3 while keeping your core strong and your arm straight against the resistance attempting to pull you back, then perform 3 quick presses. This is 1 rep. Your shoulders and hips should be facing forward. If the load is too easy to hold, step farther forward with the band. Perform 5 reps with your right arm, then switch foot positions and repeat using your left arm. You will perform a total of 15 seconds of holds and 15 presses.

**BLOCK 2**

# SANDBAG ZERCHER SQUAT

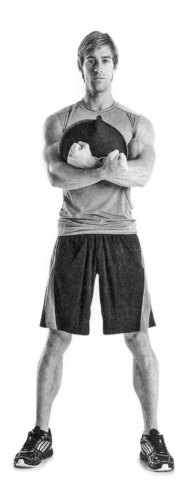
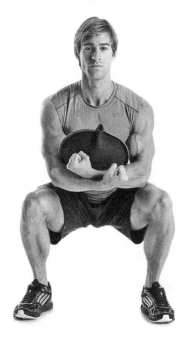

Stand, holding a sand bag or large log at chest height with your arms underneath and forearms crossed. Next, squat down while pushing your hips back as you bend your knees. The load will try to pull your torso forward, so be sure to fight to keep your body upright and locked in. Squeeze your forearms into the bag or log, pulling it toward your chest. Keep your shoulders from shrugging. Perform 12 reps using a fast tempo—take 1 second to go down, don't pause at the bottom, and push up as fast as possible with good form. Pause briefly at the top before starting the next rep.

**BLOCK 2**

# NEIDLER PRESS WITH PLATE

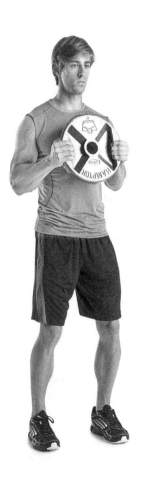 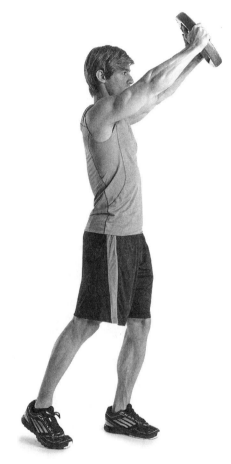

Stand with your feet shoulder-width apart, knees slightly bent. Grasp a 25- to 45-pound weight plate in your hands, gripping it like you would a steering wheel. Hold it against your chest. Now simultaneously turn your shoulders and hips left while pressing the plate away from you and pivoting on the ball of your right foot. Your arms should be extended straight and up at a 45-degree angle; your eyes should be looking through the hole in the center of the plate. Quickly return the plate to your body as you turn back to the starting position and face forward. Repeat the move, this time turning to your right and pivoting on the ball of your left foot. Do 8 reps in each direction.

## BLOCK 2

# BODYSAW

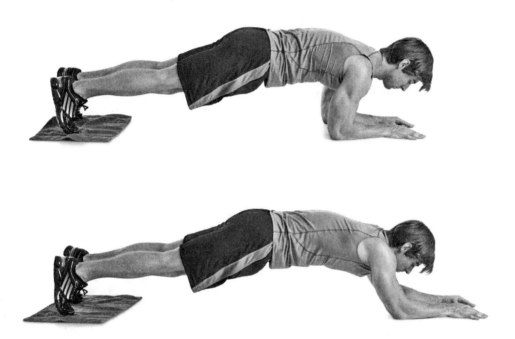

Get into a plank position with your forearms on the floor, elbows under your shoulders, head in line with your body, and feet on a face towel if you're on a hardwood floor or on glossy magazines, plastic plates, or anything that will allow your feet to slide if you're on a carpet. This is the starting position. Now, using your forearms and elbows, pull yourself forward and push yourself backward in small, controlled motions, as if your body is a saw moving back and forth to cut wood. Push yourself back just enough that your back is flat, not bowing. Stop if you feel any pain. One forward and backward motion equals 1 repetition. Do 10.

## BLOCK 2

# THE 2-MINUTE DRILL CHALLENGE

Using the original Belly Off! 2-Minute Drill, perform 10 reps each of the eight exercises below. (For alternating exercises, perform 20 total reps.) Time yourself and record your time. Rest for 60 seconds and repeat the circuit, trying to beat your first time. Each week, try to beat the previous week's best time. Every other week, reverse the order of the drill, starting with the last exercise in the list.

1. Jumping Jack
2. Prisoner Squat
3. High-Knee Skip
4. Side-to-Side Hop

5. Pushup
6. Crunch
7. Mountain Climber
8. Bodyweight Thruster (Explosive Jumps)

# Strength Workout B

This workout begins with the same strength prep exercises as Workout A, but instead of two Strength Blocks and a 2-Minute Drill circuit, you do three Strength Blocks. Complete all the exercises in each block, resting 45 seconds between exercises. Rest for 90 seconds before repeating the block. You will do two rounds before moving on to the next block. After completing all the blocks, rest for a few minutes and then walk outside to do the Hit-the-Hills Finisher, which is designed to turbocharge your metabolism and burn through serious calories. Be sure to warm up with your 2-Minute Drill, Flex Series, and even a little extra stretching for this tough workout.

# WEEKS 1 TO 3

# WORKOUT B
## WARMUP
Advanced 2-Minute Drill (see page 49) + Intermediate Flex Series (see page 89)

| STRENGTH PREP EXERCISES | REPS | SETS |
|---|---|---|
| MEDICINE BALL SCOOP TOSS | 10 | 1 |
| LATERAL SINGLE-LEG JUMP | 6 each direction | 2 |

| STRENGTH EXERCISES | REPS | SETS |
|---|---|---|
| BLOCK 1 | | |
| ISOMETRIC TOWEL DEADLIFT TO VERTICAL JUMP | 5 | 2 |
| JUMP UP/ SLOWDOWN PULLUP | 2 | 2 |
| BLOCK 2 | | |
| DUMBBELL SQUAT AND CURL | 10 | 2 |
| PUSHUP X AND ROLL | 8 | 2 |
| THREE-WAY SITUP | 6 | 2 |
| BLOCK 3 | | |
| HEAVY SUPPORTED DUMBBELL ROW | 6 each arm | 2 |
| LATERAL SUMO STEP AND PUNCH | 10 each side | 2 |
| SINGLE-LEG ROMANIAN DEADLIFT | 8 each side | 2 |
| FINISHER | | |
| HIT THE HILLS | 8 10-second runs | 1 |

# COOLDOWN
Walk (3 minutes) + Intermediate Flex Series (see page 89)

**WORKOUT B PROGRESSIONS: WEEKS 4 TO 6**
Do 3 rounds of each block

**BLOCK 1**

# ISOMETRIC TOWEL DEADLIFT TO VERTICAL JUMP

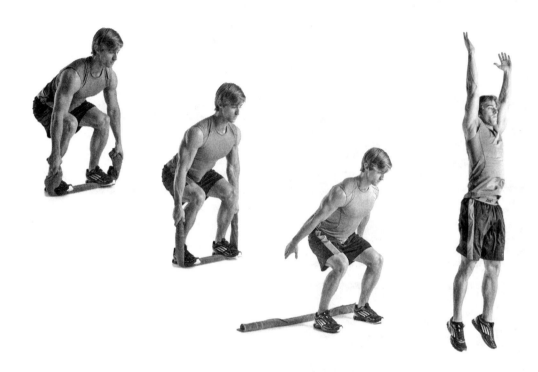

Stand on a towel or rope that's about 4 feet long, with your feet shoulder-width apart. Squat down and grasp the towel with your hands outside of your feet, your arms outside of your shins. Now push your feet through the ground and pull up on the towel for a 5-second isometric hold (keep your lower back flat to avoid injury). Release the towel, step off of it, and perform 5 quick vertical jumps: sit your hips back, knees out, and jump high, but in control. Land on the balls of your feet and allow your heels to come to the floor before leaping again. Drive your arms up to help you jump. Jump only as high as you can "stick," or control, the landing. Repeat for a total of 2 sets of this combination move, resting for 20 to 30 seconds between each round and before moving to the next exercise.

**BLOCK 1**

# JUMP UP AND
# SLOW-DOWN PULLUP

**NUTRITION**
Fuel Your
Workout

Exercise sessions that last an hour or less don't require boatloads of carbohydrates. Your muscles have enough glycogen to power at least an hour or two of moderate- to high-intensity exercise. Still, you should fuel up a little bit for even short workouts. A snack-size meal of 200 calories that includes 30 grams of carbohydrates and 20 grams of protein will do the trick. You'll get that in a sandwich made with sliced turkey breast.

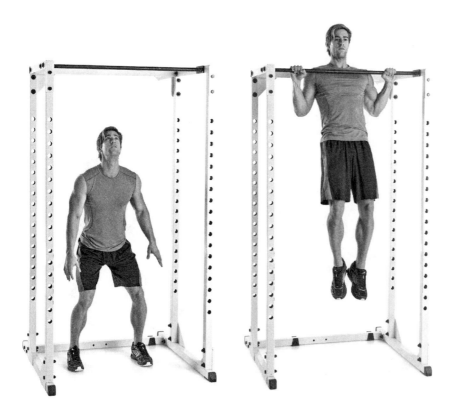

Stand under a chinup bar. Bend your knees and jump up, to allow your momentum to help you perform a pullup. Remember to pull your elbows down and back as you raise your chest to the bar. Pause for a second at the top, and then slowly lower yourself to a count of 8. Place your feet on the ground and repeat the exercise. Try to complete 2 reps, and work up to 5 by the end of 6 weeks.

**BLOCK 2**

# DUMBBELL SQUAT AND CURL

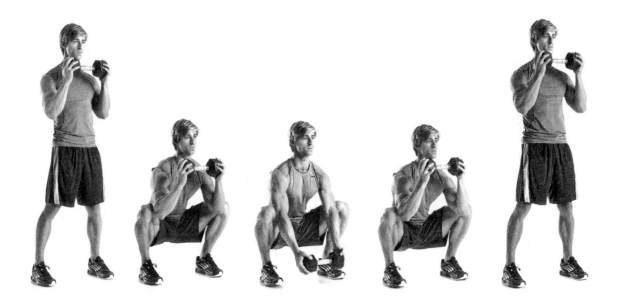

Stand with your feet about shoulder-width apart and hold one end of a dumbbell in each hand (or a kettlebell by the handle) in front of your chest. Now sit your hips back and bend your knees to perform a squat until your thighs are parallel with the ground or lower. Keeping your chest up, pause at the bottom of the squat and press your elbows against your thighs to spread your legs slightly. Next, perform a full curl and then stand up. Choose a weight that makes curl number 10 challenging but does not force you to bend forward as you stand up. Some trainers call this exercise "squat therapy" because its motion helps you fix poor squat form.

**BLOCK 2**

# PUSHUP X AND ROLL

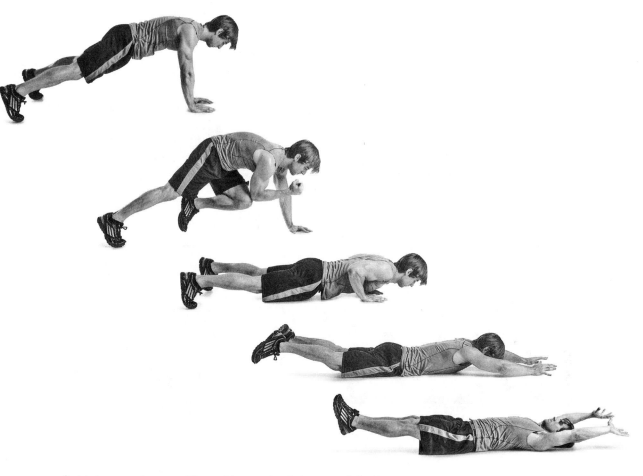

Get into a pushup position with your body in a straight line and your abs, glutes, and thighs engaged. Your hands should be directly under your shoulders. Perform a pushup. At the top, lift your right hand and left foot and bend your elbow and knee under your body until they touch. Return to the pushup position, and then touch your left elbow and right knee. That's a pushup X. Now lower yourself to the floor and complete a full-body roll to the right, ending up in the pushup position again. Press yourself up and repeat another series of the pushup X before lowering and rolling to the left. That's 1 rep. Do 8 reps.

**BLOCK 2**

# THREE-WAY SITUP

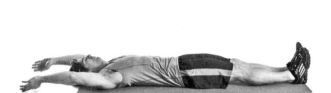

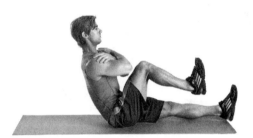

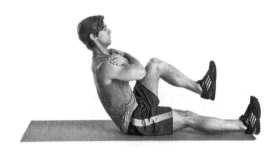

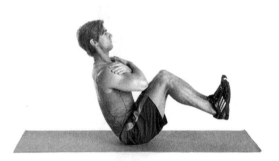

Lie flat on your back with your legs straight and your arms extended
overhead so your body forms a straight line on the floor. Now perform a
situp, sweeping your arms forward and crossing them over your chest to
give yourself a hug. While doing this, bring your right knee up to your chest.
Unfold yourself back to the starting position and repeat, this time bending
your left knee to your chest. Lie back down and this time lift both knees to
your chest as you curl up. That's one three-way repetition. Do 6 reps.

**BLOCK 3**

# HEAVY SUPPORTED DUMBBELL ROW

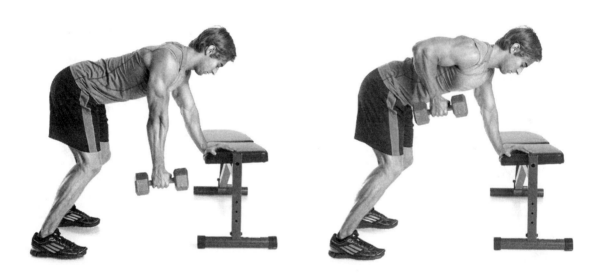

Bend over on an exercise bench with your left hand supporting you and your feet flat on the floor. Grab a heavy dumbbell with your right hand, using a neutral grip (palm facing in). Brace your abs and pull the weight up to the side of your rib cage without shrugging your shoulders or rotating your torso. Return to the starting position. That's 1 rep. Do 6 reps, switch sides, and perform 6 reps on the other side.

**BLOCK 3**

# LATERAL SUMO STEP AND PUNCH

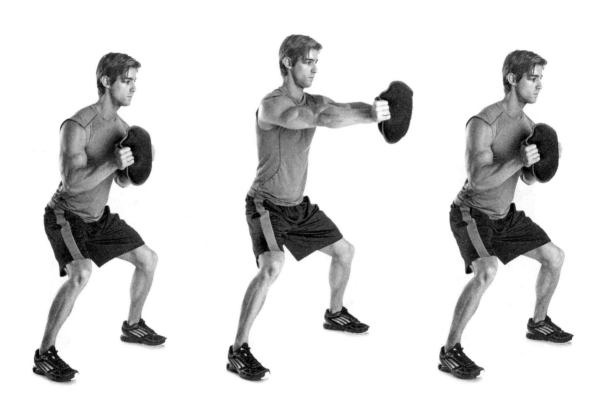

Hold a dumbbell, sandbag, or weight plate by both ends in your hands in front of your chest. With your knees bent, hips back, chest up, and feet twice as wide as shoulder-width apart, with toes pointing slightly out, step laterally with your right leg as you press the dumbbell away from your chest until your arms are straight out in front of you. Staying low, step in with your right foot to the starting position (sumo-style squat stance) as you pull the weight back to your chest. Repeat for 10 steps to the right and then 10 steps to the left. Don't let your feet come together, and keep your head level.

## BLOCK 3

# SINGLE-LEG
# ROMANIAN DEADLIFT

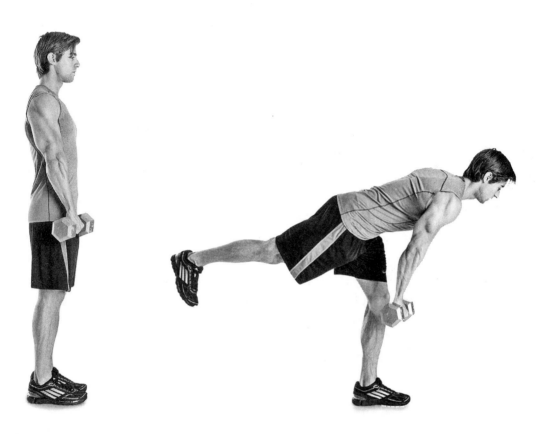

Stand with your feet hip-width apart. Holding a dumbbell with your right
hand in front of your thigh, bend at your waist, keeping a flat back. Raise
your right foot and extend it behind you. Contract your glutes, brace your
abs, and keep your spine naturally arched. Focusing on balance, lower
yourself forward until your torso is parallel to the floor; allow your back
leg to rise to parallel with the floor as a counterbalance. Initiate the
movement by pushing your hips back. Pause for 2 or 3 seconds, then push
back up to the starting position. That's 1 rep. Do 8 reps, then perform
another 8 reps holding the weight in your left hand and balancing on your
right foot.

## BLOCK 3: FINISHER

# HIT THE HILLS

Find a moderately steep hill. (You could also use stairs or bleacher steps at a stadium, or even a treadmill set to a steep incline.) Run "uphill" for 10 seconds as hard as you can. Rest to recover and repeat the sequence 7 more times. With each subsequent rep, try to run farther than you did the previous rep. Rest for no longer than 60 seconds between reps. Time yourself. Each week, seek to improve your time.

# Strength Workout C

We call this workout Everything But the Kitchen Sink because that's what we're going to throw at you. It's a jumble of new moves designed to confuse and challenge your muscles. Today's workout is also multiplanar and "functional" in nature, with your hips, shoulders, knees, and spine all being forced to move quickly in various ways. The loads are light, but the intensity isn't. The workout is up-tempo, so crank the appropriate tunes, if you're so inclined. Move steadily and pay attention to your form. Get it done, and have fun!

### CORE PREP

Do 1 set of the following exercises, resting 30 seconds after each exercise and 1 minute between rounds. Perform 2 rounds.

- Anti-Rotation Press Out
- Overhead Band "Soccer" Throw-In
- Glute Bridge (see page 37)
- Turtle
- Back Extension

## SUCCESS STORY

# Make Exercise Part of Your Lifestyle

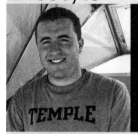

**Weight Before**

# 236

**Weight After**

# 174

## BRYN DAVIS

HORSHAM, PA
THE BELLY OFF! CLUB, SEPTEMBER 2010

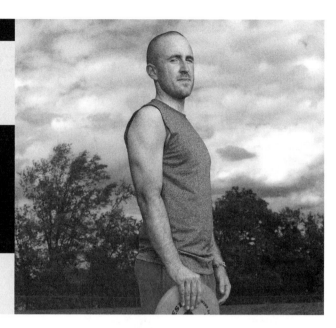

### THE WAKE-UP CALL

I used to eat like a glutton—anything I wanted, in vast quantities—and yet I was lean and strong because I was on my high school's crew team. Then I went to college and didn't play sports. But I did keep up my eating. Maybe I ate even more because, hey, it was there for the taking. Two years in, I wasn't feeling well. I had bad skin. My hair looked unhealthy. I tired quickly. And I was avoiding some social situations because I'd lost confidence in how I looked. College was passing me by.

At home on break during my junior year of college, I went for my annual doctor's visit. I stood on his scale and was blown away: 236 pounds! My weight had been in the low 170s in high school. I'd heard of the freshman 15— but the freshman 60-plus? I was able to ignore my weight before, but now I was scared into action.

### HOW I CHANGED

I was always a mass-consumption kind of guy, so I had to find healthier ways to fill up. Fiber was the key: Now I always eat oatmeal in the morning, and I snack on a Fiber One bar and a tall glass of water during the day. Another snack I like is popcorn with a little sea salt, cayenne, and Old Bay seasoning. I was never big on fruits, but I enjoy them in a meal-replacement smoothie once or twice a day. My favorite: frozen blueberry and pineapple with a little agave nectar and a base of almond milk.

I transferred to another college and befriended a group of wrestlers. Being around healthy guys motivated me to work out. I started with the elliptical machine because it wasn't overwhelming and it tracked how many calories I burned. When I dropped to under 200 pounds, I hit the weights hard. I'd do cardio for an hour a day, and mix up the weightlifting 5 or 6 days a week. My regular gym visit stopped feeling like a chore and started feeling like part of my lifestyle.

### THE REWARD

Everything looks and feels healthier, even my hair and skin. The weight loss has been so life-changing that I opened up a healthy quick-service food shop near Philly that serves as an alternative to regular fast-food joints. I'm on a mission to share what I've learned with others so they can feel as good as I do now.

CORE PREP

# ANTI-ROTATION PRESS OUT

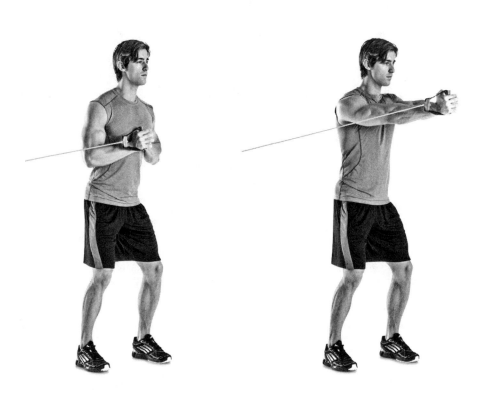

Stand perpendicular to an adjustable cable stack with your right side facing the cable machine and your feet hip-width apart. Grasp the cable handle with your left hand and wrap your right hand over your left. Bring the handle to the middle of your chest, raising the weight stack. This is the starting position. Now press the handle forward and tense your core to resist the tension pulling you toward the cable stack. Hold your hands outstretched for 3 seconds, then bring the handle back to your chest. That's 1 rep. Perform 5 reps, then switch sides and do 5 more reps. Be sure that the hand to the side wraps over the hand on the handle. If you don't have a cable machine, you can do this exercise with exercise tubing anchored to a stationary object.

CORE PREP

# OVERHEAD BAND "SOCCER" THROW-IN

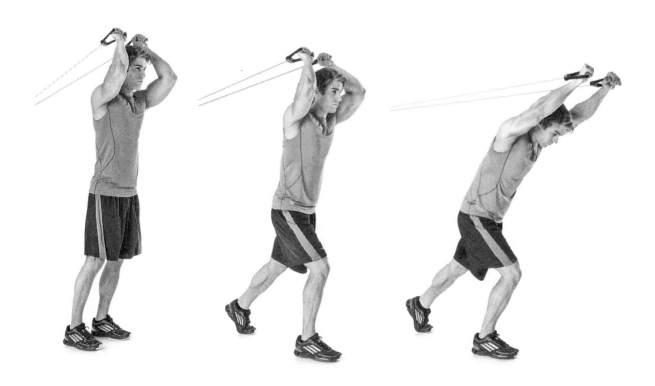

Anchor an exercise band to a secure object at chest height. Grasp the handles of the band with both hands and turn your back toward the anchor, lifting your hands behind your head. Step forward to create tension in the band. Don't arch your back. This is the starting position. Lean slightly forward, take a step, and straighten your arms as if throwing a soccer ball over your head. Allow the band to pull your hands back over your head and repeat the "toss" for a total of 12 reps while alternating the lead leg each time.

## CORE PREP

# TURTLE

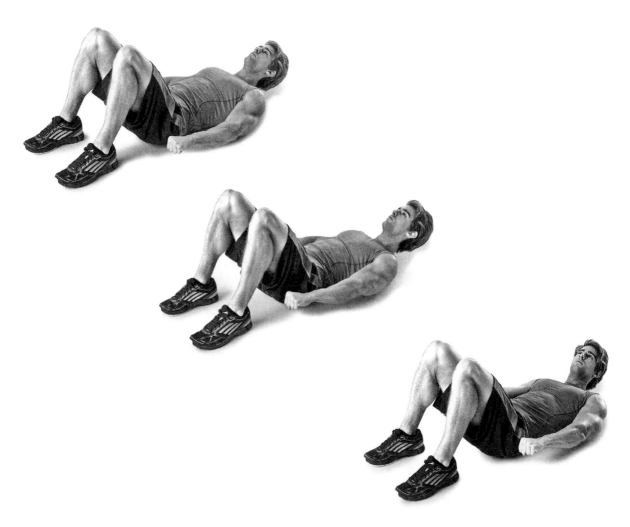

Lie on your back with your knees bent, arms at your sides, and feet flat on the ground. Perform a small isometric crunch, driving your belly button toward your spine and squeezing your abs. While holding this position (with a relaxed neck), slide your straight right arm slowly toward your right heel and return to start. Perform the same move on the left side. This is 1 rep. Perform 16 reps.

## CORE PREP

# BACK EXTENSION

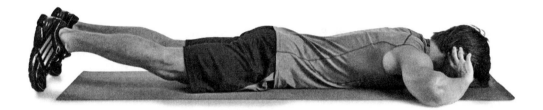

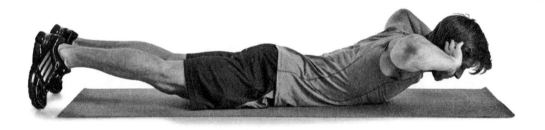

Lie facedown on the floor and place your hands lightly on the sides of your head. Keeping your hips pressed into the floor, toes on the ground, and glutes clenched, pull your chest a few inches off the floor by squeezing your upper back and lifting it toward the ceiling. Pause at the top for a count of 1, then lower your body to the floor. Perform 10 reps. If you feel pain in your low back, try reducing your range of motion. If the move still hurts, stop.

# Strength Workout C

There are three circuits in this workout. Follow the prescribed order for each week.

**Week 1:** Perform the circuits in order; do 2 rounds of each circuit before advancing to the next circuit.

**Week 2:** Perform the circuits in reverse order (not including the finisher); do 2 rounds of each circuit before advancing to the next circuit.

**Weeks 3 through 6:** Perform the circuits in order, one exercise after the other, completing all 10 of the exercises in a row in a giant round. Rest as needed between exercises and up to 90 seconds between rounds. Perform 2 giant rounds. Repeat the same cycle for weeks 3 through 5, and simply increase the last workout on Week 6 to 3 rounds to finish strong!

# WORKOUT C
## WARMUP

Advanced 2-Minute Drill (page 49)
Intermediate Flex Series (page 89)

| CORE PREP EXERCISES | REPS | SETS |
|---|---|---|
| ANTI-ROTATION PRESS OUT | 5 each side | 1 |
| OVERHEAD BAND "SOCCER" THROW-IN | 12 | 1 |
| GLUTE BRIDGE | 10 | 1 |
| TURTLE | 16 | 1 |
| BACK EXTENSION | 10 | 1 |

| STRENGTH EXERCISES | REPS | ROUNDS |
|---|---|---|
| CIRCUIT 1 | | 2 |
| ½ TURKISH GETUP | 3 with each arm | |
| DUMBBELL SWING AND STEP | 10 with each leg | |
| ALTERNATING DUMBBELL PRESS | 8 | |
| CIRCUIT 2 | | 2 |
| DUMBBELL REVERSE LUNGE/CHOP | 8 to each side | |
| DUMBBELL SINGLE-ARM PRESS, ON KNEE | 8 with each arm | |
| STANDING BAND SPEED ROW | As many as possible in 10 seconds | |
| CIRCUIT 3 | | 2 |
| LATERAL CROSSOVER STEPUP | 60 seconds | |
| BURDENKO RUSSIAN DANCE | 45 seconds | |
| THREE-WAY PLANK FOOT TOUCH | As many as possible in 30 seconds | |
| BENCH HURDLE AND RUN | 5 to each side | |
| FINISHER: THE ALL-STAR ATHLETE | | 1 |
| THE JUMP SHOT | 16 | |
| THE BOWLER | 6 to each side | |
| THE LINEMAN | 30 seconds | |
| THE ARCHER | 5 to each side | |
| THE JUKE | 10 | |

## COOLDOWN

Walk (3 minutes)
Intermediate Flex Series (see page 89)

## CIRCUIT 1

# ½ TURKISH GETUP

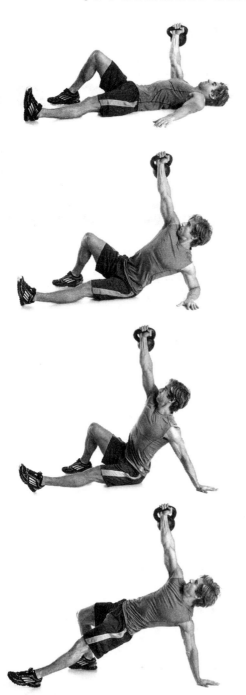

Grab a dumbbell or kettlebell in your right hand and lie with your back on the floor, your right knee bent and your right foot flat on the ground. Raise the weight over your right shoulder with your arm extended. Your left leg should be straight and your left arm should be at a 45-degree angle to your body, palm facing down. This is the starting position. Now, using your core, turn your body toward the left as you push the weight up and work to move onto your left elbow and forearm by drawing that arm toward you. (You will be rotating your torso to the left while keeping your left leg on the floor.) Next, push the weight straight up and even higher as you work to extend your left arm straight and support yourself with your left hand flat on the floor. Finally, bridge up by pressing your right leg and foot and left hand through the floor to raise your butt off the floor. Squeeze your right glute and hold this bridge position for a count of 3. Slowly reverse the steps back down to the starting position. Perform a total of 3 reps on one side before repeating the move on the opposite side. The trick to doing this exercise properly is to do it slowly and under control, one step at a time, always keeping the load up under a straight arm and always keeping your eyes on the weight.

**CIRCUIT 1**

# DUMBBELL SWING AND STEP

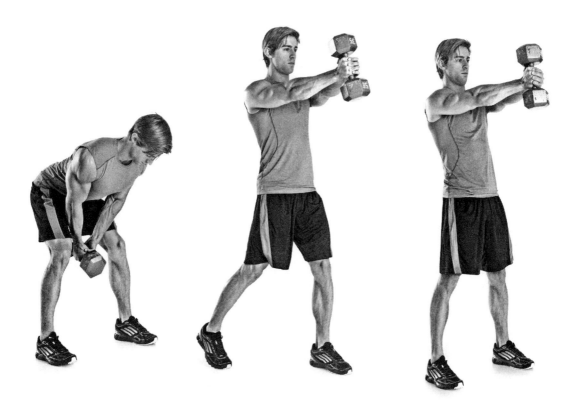

Hold a single dumbbell with both hands interlaced around the handle. Stand with your feet shoulder-width apart, bend at the waist, and allow the dumbbell to hang between your legs. This is the starting position. Now, keeping your arms straight, swing the dumbbell up and away from your body, using your hips as the primary driver as you stand. As the dumbbell swings up, step backward with your right foot and plant it as the weight reaches its apex in front of your eyes. Push through your left foot and step up with your right foot parallel with your left as the dumbbell starts to swing back down. Alternate feet with each step and swing. Your chest should be up, eyes forward, and knee slightly bent as your forward leg lands. The move should be fluid. If it's not, try using a lighter dumbbell. Perform 20 reps alternating legs.

**CIRCUIT 1**

# ALTERNATING DUMBBELL PRESS

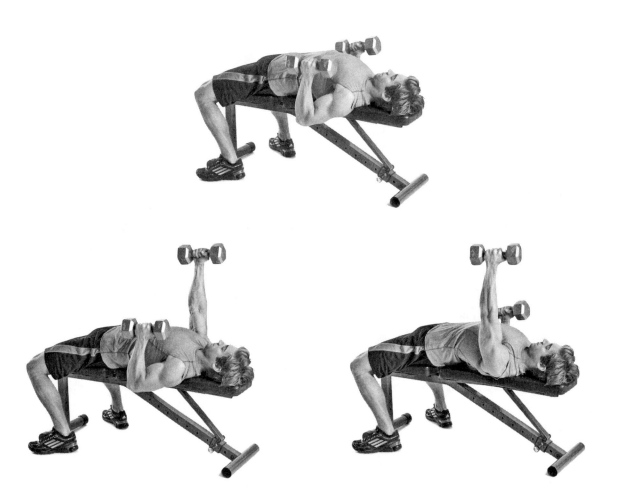

Grab two dumbbells and lie on a bench with your feet on the floor and your hips, shoulders, and head in contact with the bench. Lower the dumbbells to your armpits and hold them just slightly off of your chest, so they do not rest on your body. This is the starting position. Without rotating your body, press one dumbbell away from your body until your arm is extended. Return it to the bottom position, and then press the dumbbell in the other hand. That's 1 rep. Continue alternating this way for 8 reps.

**CIRCUIT 2**

# DUMBBELL REVERSE LUNGE/CHOP

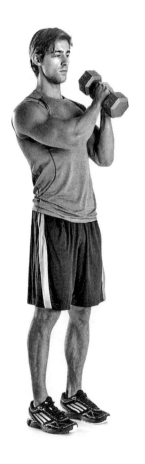
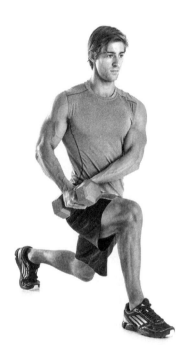

Hold one dumbbell in your hands with your fingers interlaced around the handle. Hold the weight at your left shoulder. Step backward with your left leg into a reverse lunge as you swing the dumbbell down toward your right hip, bracing your core and keeping your torso upright. Keep the dumbbell at your right hip as you stand up. On the next rep, as you lunge backward with your left foot, raise the dumbbell from your right hip to your left shoulder. Keep it there as you stand back up. That's 1 rep. Perform 8 reps, then switch sides and repeat the exercise on the other side (lunging back with your right leg, dumbbell moving from right shoulder to left hip).

**CIRCUIT 2**

# DUMBBELL SINGLE-ARM PRESS, ON A KNEE

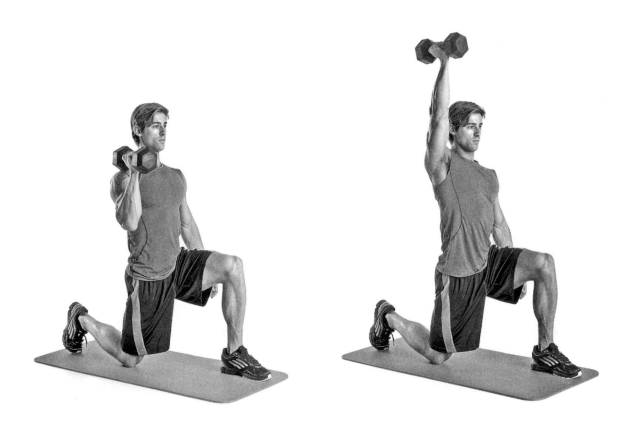

Hold a dumbbell in your right hand and kneel on your right knee. (You may place a pillow or towel under your knee for comfort.) Position your knee slightly behind your hip and bring your left leg forward, foot flat on the floor and shin nearly vertical. Lift the dumbbell to your shoulder, palm facing inward. This is the starting position. Now, press the dumbbell overhead until your right arm is fully extended, making sure to keep your biceps near your ear and your chest up as you press the weight. Lower the weight to your shoulder. That's 1 rep. After completing 8 reps on that side, switch sides and repeat.

**CIRCUIT 2**

# STANDING BAND SPEED ROW

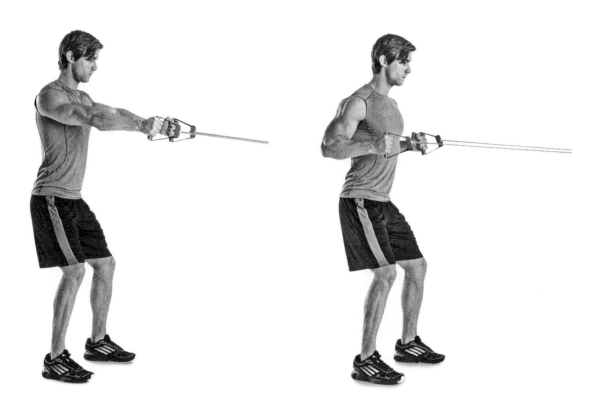

Anchor the middle of an exercise band to a stationary object at chest height. Grasp a handle in each hand, face the anchor, and step backward to create tension on the band. Stand with your feet shoulder-width apart, knees slightly bent. This is the starting position. Now, quickly pull your fists toward your lower rib cage and extend your arms back out; continue this in-and-out for 10 seconds, performing as many reps as possible. Rest for 10 seconds. That's 1 round. Do 2 more rounds. Don't rotate your body, curl your wrists, or shrug your shoulders.

### CIRCUIT 3

# LATERAL CROSSOVER STEPUP

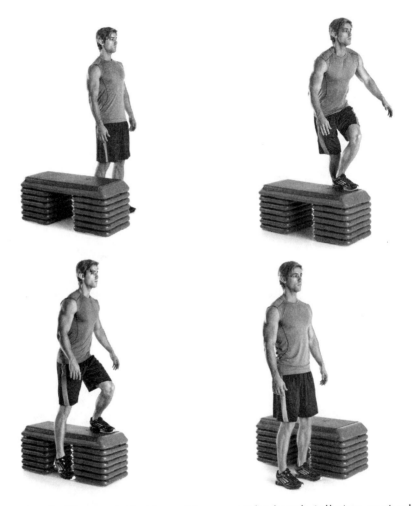

Stand with your right side next to an exercise bench, tall step, or sturdy box that's about 18 inches tall. Lift your left leg across your body and onto the bench. Press through your left foot to raise your body up and across the bench. Your right leg should follow your body over the bench; land your right foot on the ground in control, and bend at your hips and knee to absorb the force of the landing. Immediately bring your left leg off the bench so you are standing with the bench to your left side. Repeat, moving in the other direction, and continue alternating reps for 60 seconds.

## CIRCUIT 3

# BURDENKO RUSSIAN DANCE

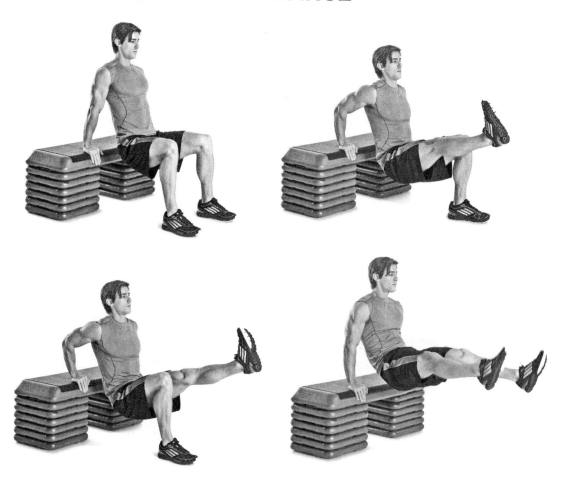

Sit on a bench, step, or armless chair. Place both hands behind you on the bench and lower your body as if to perform a triceps dip with your back against the bench. Your knees should be bent and both feet flat on the ground. Pushing your back away from the bench, extend one leg out and away from your body, as if to flick the foot away, return it quickly, extend the other leg and return it, and then, jumping up, extend both legs. Alternate your lead leg while performing this single-leg, single-leg, double-leg pattern for 45 seconds. The movement should be fluid, dynamic, and have some up and down motion.

### CIRCUIT 3

# THREE-WAY PLANK FOOT TOUCH

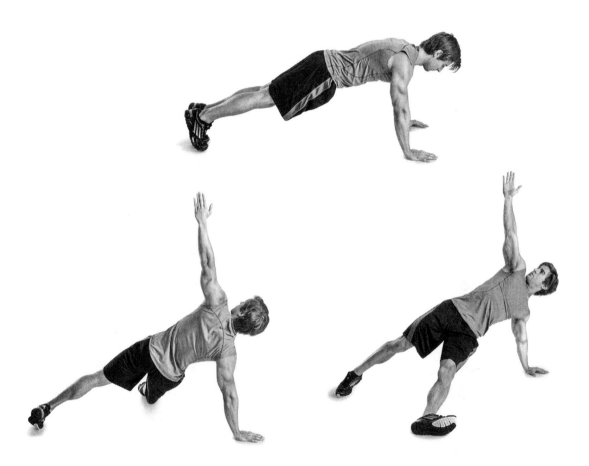

Get into a pushup position on your toes, with your arms straight, hands on the ground directly underneath your shoulders, and back straight from heels to head. This is position 1. Next, drive your right leg toward your left side, keeping it straight as you rotate your body open, raising your left hand toward the ceiling. Return your leg and hand to position 1. Drive your left leg toward your right side, rising your right hand toward the ceiling. As soon as you tap your heel, return to position 1 and quickly repeat the three-step movement as many times as you can in 30 seconds. Be sure to keep your body—head to heel—as strong as steel throughout the movement.

**CIRCUIT 3**

# BENCH HURDLE AND RUN

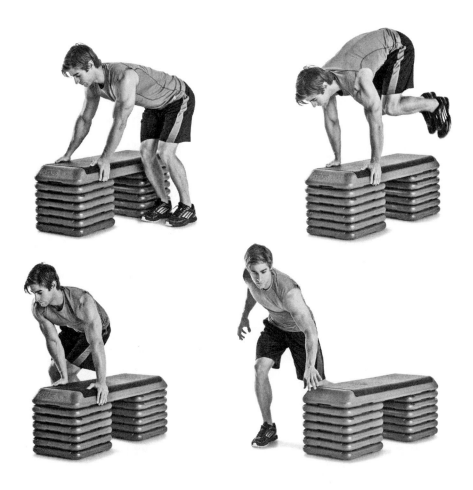

Stand with an exercise bench on your right side and place both hands on it. Keeping your hands on the bench, bend your knees and jump laterally over the bench. When your feet touch the ground, immediately run forward a few steps, then step two steps to your left, then step backward until you are back in the starting position. Place your hands on the bench again, and repeat the jump and run. Do 5 repetitions one way, and then switch sides and perform 5 more going the other way and around the back of the bench. Rest 90 seconds before doing another round.

### FINISHER: THE ALL-STAR ATHLETE

Perform the following circuit one time, as quickly as possible with good form. Seek to beat your time each week.

# THE JUMP SHOT

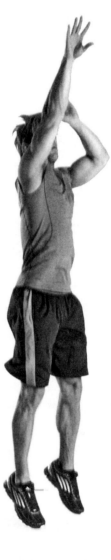

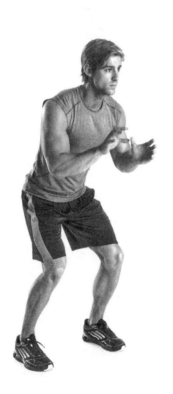

Stand with feet hip-width apart, and then step to one side and jump in the air as if to take a jump shot. Land softly, step to the other side, and repeat. Perform 16 jump shots. As an added bonus, follow through with your hands.

## FINISHER: THE ALL-STAR ATHLETE

# THE BOWLER

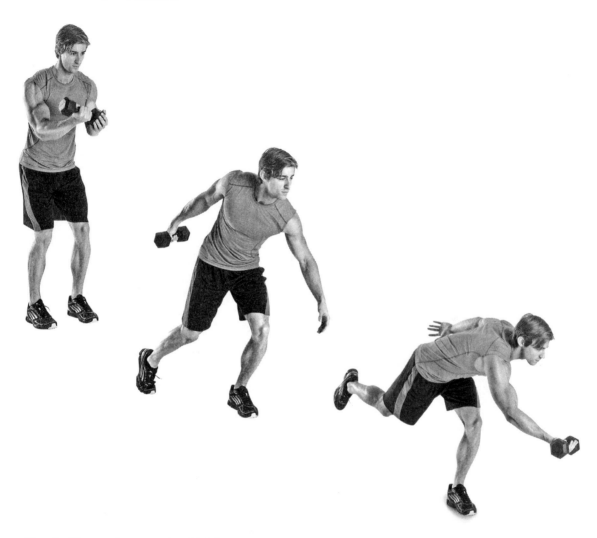

Stand with your feet together. Holding a light (5-pound) dumbbell in your right hand, step forward with your left foot, and swing the dumbbell back and forward, as if launching a bowling ball. (But don't let go of the dumbbell!) Pause for a count of 1 at the "release," with both legs bent as in a lunge position and your body low. Return to the starting position. That's 1 rep. Do 6 reps, switch sides, and repeat for 6 reps.

## FINISHER: THE ALL-STAR ATHLETE

# THE LINEMAN

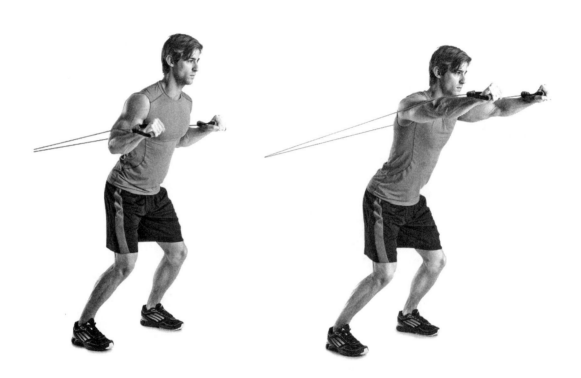

Attach exercise bands to a secure object or use a cable station. Hold a band or cable handle in each hand and step forward to create resistance. Stand with your feet shoulder-width apart and your knees slightly bent. Lean forward slightly so the bands or cables pull your hands to the sides of your chest. Now bend forward a bit more and press your arms out in front of you as if pushing a rushing defensive lineman off of you. Hold this isometric position for 30 seconds. The resistance should be heavy enough that you really have to drive your feet into the floor and anchor your core to avoid being pulled backward.

## FINISHER: THE ALL-STAR ATHLETE

# THE ARCHER

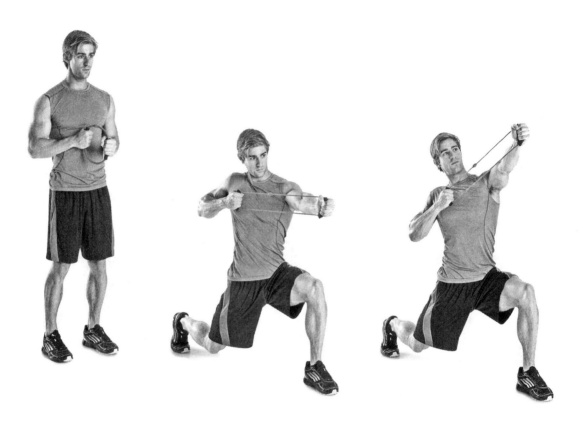

Hold one end of a resistance band in both hands in front of you at chest height. Stand with feet hip-width apart facing forward, and then take a step backward into a reverse lunge with your right foot and pull the band toward your armpit as you extend your opposite arm, just as if you were drawing back an arrow with your right hand and holding a bow with your left. Pause here for a count of 2, then extend your lead arm up toward the ceiling and in front of you at a 45-degree angle, pausing here for a count of 2. Return your arms to straight as you stand up. That's 1 rep. Perform 5 reps on one side, switch sides, and repeat for 5 more.

## FINISHER: THE ALL-STAR ATHLETE

# THE JUKE

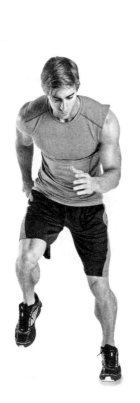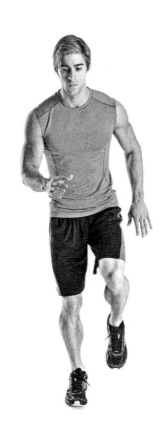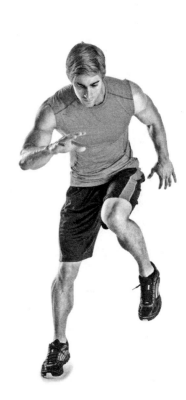

Stand with your feet about hip-width apart, knees slightly bent. Shuffle 2 steps to your left—step, together, step, together—and raise your right leg off the ground as you plant your left leg on the second step. Immediately shuffle 2 steps to your right, raising your left leg off the ground as you plant your right foot on the second step. That's 1 rep. Do 10 reps total. Do not allow your body to lean to the side that you are stopping on, and seek to "juke" the defender who might be trying to stop you.

# ADVANCED CARDIO WORKOUTS

You'll perform 3 different cardio workouts per week—2 high-intensity interval days, 1 steady-state aerobic day, and at least 1 fun fitness play day. Do your interval workouts on the days when you aren't doing a strength training workout. Remember to warm up with a Belly Off! Advanced 2-Minute Drill and the Flex Series.

## INTERVAL DAY 1

For Interval Day 1, you can run, bike, swim, or use indoor cardio equipment. It's your choice, but try to change up your activity every week during the 6-week program. As you know, intervals are quick bursts of fast-paced intense exercise followed by short bouts of slow recovery movement. This workout is 15 minutes for Week 1. Add 1 minute more to each subsequent week.

Every other week, you will switch between two different interval patterns (A and B) for Interval Day 1 (see the chart below).

**Pattern A:** 10 seconds of running at an effort level of 8 on a scale of 1 to 10, followed by 10 seconds of recovery, followed by 10 seconds of level-8 running, followed by 30 seconds of recovery at an exertion level of 3 or 4. Repeat this pattern until the last 3 minutes of your workout, when you should cool down by gradually decreasing your speed to a walk.

**Pattern B:** Alternate these two patterns every minute:

- 20 seconds on (effort level 8), 40 seconds off (recovery level 4)
- 5 seconds on (effort level 8), 15 seconds off (recovery level 4), repeated 3 times.

After Week 1, add 1 minute of exercise time to each workout.

| WEEK | 1 | 2 | 3 | 4 | 5 | 6 |
|------|---|---|---|---|---|---|
| TIME | 15 minutes | 16 minutes | 17 minutes | 18 minutes | 19 minutes | 20 minutes |
| PATTERN | A | B | A | B | A | B for 10 minutes and A for 10 minutes |

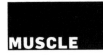

## MUSCLE
Parched Tongue, Low T

Drink water before your strength session. According to a 2008 study in the *Journal of Applied Physiology*, dehydration causes men to produce more of the stress hormone cortisol during strength training, and it reduces the release of the muscle-building hormone testosterone.

## INTERVAL DAY 2

For Interval Day 2, you'll perform shuttles on a grassy surface or running track. To do this, set up two markers 25 yards apart. Run out and back as fast as possible—that's 1 rep. Follow the reps and rest schedule below. Time yourself and record it.

**Week 1:** 3 reps, rest for 90 seconds, repeat 2 more times
**Week 2:** 3 reps, rest for 75 seconds, repeat 3 more times
**Week 3:** 4 reps, rest for 75 seconds, repeat 3 more times
**Week 4:** 6 reps, rest for 120 seconds, repeat 2 more times
**Week 5:** 6 reps, rest for 120 seconds, repeat 3 more times
**Week 6:** 3 reps, rest for 60 seconds, repeat 5 more times

## STEADY-STATE AEROBIC DAY

Choose a trail or route or type of cardio equipment that's different from your interval days. Start with a 5-minute slow warmup, then increase your effort level to a 6 or 7 on an exertion scale of 1 to 10, where 10 is a sprint. At 6 or 7, you should be able to speak in a few short sentences but it shouldn't be too comfortable to talk for long. Progress as follows through the 6 weeks.

**Week 1:** Rest
**Week 2:** 30 minutes

**Week 3:** Rest
**Week 4:** 30 minutes

**Week 5:** Rest
**Week 6:** 30 minutes

## FUN FITNESS DAY

Play a sport like tennis, basketball, or softball, or go for a hike or bike ride. Do something active that you love and that involves other human beings. (Yeah, your family qualifies.) There's a good reason we recommend the group dynamic (beside the fact that it's really tough to play tennis by yourself): It'll help you live longer. Research has shown that people with few social connections live about 4½ years less than average, and one study has even suggested that being socially active can add up to a decade to your life.

# PART
# 3

## BELLY OFF! NUTRITION

When you're halfway through a box of Oreos and a carton of milk, the last thing you want to think about is what's in those delicious sandwich cookies. Reading the label would be a moot point now—and it would really bum you out.

A better plan, if you're keen on losing weight and eating healthier: not opening that box of Oreos in the first place. Keep it out of the house; in fact, leave it miles away, back in the store. Do yourself a big favor and read labels before committing to any sort of long-term relationship with packaged foods. They tend to make themselves feel right at home, and they are hard to get rid of.

When you read the success stories of Belly Off! Club members, you'll notice that nearly all of these guys made the commitment to get to know what they were putting in their mouths and found the discipline to make significant dietary changes. Exercise is important, but it's short-lived. You do much more munching than crunching over the course of the day. So cut out the big carb bombs and eat for satiety and energy (not mindlessly), and you will make remarkable progress toward taking your belly off.

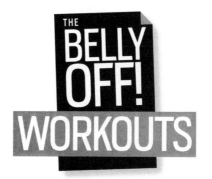

# Chapter 7

# THE BELLY OFF! DIET 6-WEEK DETOX PLAN

## Learn to Eat Clean to Lose Weight Faster and Look and Feel Healthier for Life!

L et's go on a little fact-finding mission to prove a point: Visit your pantry and find a bag of chips or a can of beef stew or any type of processed food (meaning it comes in a box, bag, carton, or can). We'll wait.

All right, now take a look at the ingredients listed on the package.

Count 'em. Are there 4, 10, 12? How many of those tidbits can you identify? How many of those do you have trouble even pronouncing?

Not to pick on any particular product, but the ingredient count on our bag of Doritos Blazin' Buffalo and Ranch Tortilla Chips, pilfered from one of our kids (*shhhh . . .* ), topped 36. Thirty-six! Where'd they put all that stuff?

We also have a tub of natural peanut butter—or what's left of it—sitting here. The ingredients list on the back reads: peanuts.

The point is, when you buy fresh-ground roasted peanut butter (not the mass-produced kind with added sugar, oil, and preservatives), you're getting pureed peanuts and nothing more. But with the chips, you're getting a whole lot more than corn— not the least of which is a set of orange fingers. It's the same for any processed food product, whether you bring it home from the grocery store or order it through the window of your car. It's just loaded with all kinds of manufactured stuff.

How long have you been eating that way? For most of us, the answer is: "All of our lives." It's scary when you realize that some of the things you've eaten sound like they belong in toilet bowl cleaner, not soft drinks.

The Belly Off! Diet 6-Week Detox Plan is a jumping-off point for a healthier way of eating that will help you to achieve the quickest and most impressive results from the Belly Off! workouts. We call this plan a detox, but don't worry—it has nothing to do with colonics. We're talking about rebooting your body by making cleaner food choices, not by irrigating your bowels. The Belly Off! Diet 6-Week Detox Plan is designed to help wean you off of processed foods that are loaded with sugar, fat, sodium, and chemical additives.

"Unfortunately, these are staples in the American diet that can and do lead to weight gain, high blood pressure, diabetes, heart disease, and premature aging," says sports nutritionist

Chris Mohr, PhD, RD, who helped us develop this detox plan to use along with the Belly Off! workouts. If you're a member of our online Belly Off! Club, you'll be familiar with this name because Dr. Mohr is the Belly Off! nutritionist, and he writes a popular nutrition blog at menshealth.com/bellyoff. He is a registered dietician, weight-loss expert, and sports nutrition consultant to the Cincinnati Bengals, and a founder of mohrresults.com.

The 6-week detox includes the core principles of the Belly Off! diet (regular fueling, replacing processed carbs with foods that won't spike your blood sugar, drinking more water, cutting out alcohol), but the detox goes even further. It provides more prescriptive detail for those who want to dedicate extra effort to improving their diet through a more structured approach.

If you don't want to mess around with calorie, protein, and fiber goals, you can simply commit to the nutrition promises in the Belly Off! Club Code of Conduct (on page xvi) and still achieve amazing results. However, by following the 12 rules, starting on page 176, for the same 6 weeks that you tackle the Belly Off! workout program, you'll set yourself up for the greatest weight loss and muscle gain. Even more important, you'll have your best opportunity to change deep-seated eating habits. You'll feel such a boost in energy and mental clarity by eating good stuff and eliminating junk that you'll never want to go back to your old ways.

**MOTIVATION**
## Give Yourself a Sign

Stick a note of encouragement on your bathroom mirror, refrigerator, or steering wheel to remind you to stick to your 12-point detox plan. One study showed that signs posted at a workplace to urge people to take the stairs increased stair usage by 200 percent.

# THE 6-WEEK BELLY OFF! DETOX NUTRITION PLAN

Have you signed and dated your Belly Off! Club Code of Conduct promise? Have you taken your "before" snapshot and taped it to your refrigerator as a reminder to keep your paws off that bottle of Dogfish Head ale? Have you stepped on the scale and recorded your weight? Have you told your mother so she could harp on

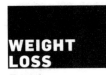

you about getting back in shape? (Accountability counts, remember?)

Good—then you're prepared for the next 6 weeks of life-changing, diet-overhauling, belly-shedding fun. Here's the point-to-point Belly Off! diet road map that Dr. Mohr recommends you team with your 6-week Belly Off! fitness plan.

## POINT #1: PICK A GOAL WEIGHT AND FIND YOUR DAILY CALORIE GOAL.

We want being healthy and looking and feeling good to be your idea of success, but the fact of the matter is that specific goals help to motivate. Keeping your eye on a prize will reinforce your will to adhere to all of the rules that follow. (Besides, choosing a realistic goal weight is necessary for the second half of this point.) Your goal weight should be the weight you wish to be for life and not reflective of the weight loss you hope to achieve at the end of only 6 weeks. Do you have a number in mind? Good. Now you need to figure out your daily calorie goal. We're not asking you to weigh your food or count the calories in each bite you take—the purpose of this goal is just to make you more aware of the calories in foods and how they affect your weight and energy. Your daily calorie goal is an approximate number that will remind you to control your portions and select those foods that are naturally low in calories and high in water, fiber, and nutrients.

To find your ballpark daily calorie goal, multiply your goal weight in pounds by 10. If, for example, your goal weight is 195 pounds, your daily calorie goal would be 1,950, or roughly 2,000 calories.

Again, do your best to tally your calories, but don't stress out if your number crunching doesn't impress your CPA or bookie. Many of the rules that follow will *automatically* keep your daily calories in check, especially Points 9 and 10, which work like magic.

# Calculate Your Calorie and Nutrient Goals

| FOOD | CURRENT BODY WEIGHT | GOAL BODY WEIGHT | X FACTOR | YOUR GOAL INTAKE FOR THE DAY |
|------|---------------------|------------------|----------|------------------------------|
| Calories | | | **x 10** | = _____ calories |
| Carbohydrates | | | **x 1** | = _____ g |
| Protein | | | **x 1** | = _____ g |
| Fat | | | **x 0.25** | = _____ g |
| Water | | | **x 0.50** | = _____ ounces |

## POINT #2: CUT OUT FAST-FOOD MEALS.

Cook more. Eat out less. You'll save about 500 calories every day that you don't eat at a fast-food restaurant. Here's another reason to avoid the drive-thru: Eating fast food just twice a week is linked to higher blood sugar levels and insulin resistance, according to an Australian study.

## POINT #3: EMBRACE MONOTONY.

Be a boring lunch eater. That's right. One easy way to cut down on calories is to have the same healthy, low-calorie lunch every day: A big salad of greens and vegetables with grilled chicken on top. A turkey or egg-salad sandwich and some sliced red peppers. Make lunch fast, simple, and the same every day. The more you complicate things, the more food choices you have available, the more likely you are to step out of the measured routine of healthy eating and into the fast-food lane. A visit to an all-you-can-eat buffet in Vegas will provide anecdotal evidence that variety leads to bigger guts, but if you want real science . . . have you heard about the M&M experiment? This is a classic by Brian Wansink, PhD, director of the Food and

Brand Lab at Cornell University. In his study, a group of about 100 people were presented with bowls of M&M candies to snack on while watching TV. They were free to eat as much as they wanted. Nobody would judge them. But the bowls were not all the same. Some contained M&M's in 10 different colors, while others contained only 7 different colors, although all the bowls contained the same total number of individual candies. The experiment revealed what Wansink expected: The people who ate from the bowls containing a greater variety of colors of M&M's consumed more M&M's. Wansink says our eyes are drawn to more variety and our brains find variety more appealing, so we eat more. The experiment showed that it's not only the variety but also the *perception* of variety that triggers us to eat more.

## POINT #4: GET SERIOUS ABOUT EATING MORE FRUITS AND VEGETABLES.

Make these your primary sources of carbohydrates and you'll automatically eat less bread, pasta, and rice—and automatically lose weight.

Each day, aim to eat 1 gram of carbohydrates from fruits or vegetables per pound of your goal body weight. For example, if your goal weight is 195 pounds, you should aim for 195 grams of carbs from fruits, vegetables, and beans each day. The nice thing about eating a smaller variety of foods each week—like the same lunch every day—is that you won't have to think much about counting grams of any of the macronutrients. Still, it's not very hard to eyeball your daily carb quota. A medium-size apple delivers about 15 grams of carbohydrates, a 1-cup serving of broccoli florets contains 10 grams, a ½-cup serving of black beans provides about 20 grams. Since a serving of most fruits and vegetables delivers between 10 and 25 grams of carbs, a man with a goal weight of 190 should shoot for roughly 8 to 12 servings. A woman with a goal weight of 145 pounds should shoot for 7 to 10. That's probably a good deal more than you are eating now, which is the very reason we've made this Point #4.

## POINT #5: TRY TO EAT 1 GRAM OF PROTEIN PER POUND OF YOUR GOAL BODY WEIGHT.

Protein fills you up. It keeps you from running to the candy machine at 3 p.m. And it builds calorie-burning muscle. If you eat enough protein, you'll automatically lower your intake of carbs, especially those that boost blood sugar.

If your goal weight is 185 pounds, that means you have a daily goal of 185 grams of protein. You're probably not eating that much daily. But if you do—just as with eating more vegetables—you'll automatically cut down on fast-burning carbohydrates. The protein will satisfy you better and longer. Eating more protein takes a little planning, but it's not that difficult if you shoot for making protein a part of every meal and snack. Here are some simple examples.

- Two eggs for breakfast: 35 grams.
- A part-skim cheese stick and a handful of almonds: 16 grams.
- A turkey and cheese sandwich: about 20 grams.
- A steak and black bean burrito: about 60 grams.
- A peanut butter and skim milk shake made with two scoops of whey protein powder: 54 grams.

## POINT #6: AIM FOR 0.25 GRAMS OF HEALTHY FATS PER POUND OF YOUR GOAL BODY WEIGHT.

Fat has been maligned as bad for your health and heart. But in reality, it's a very important part of a healthy diet. Fat aids in digestion. It transports important fat-soluble vitamins A, D, E, and K. And it provides essential fatty acids that your body can't manufacture. Most Americans would do well to be more concerned with limiting calories than reducing fat. Eating fat can actually help you trim calories. Studies show that eating fat triggers the release of a hormone that promotes feelings of satiety. If your goal weight is between 145 and 190 pounds, you should shoot for 40 to 55 grams of fat per day.

## POINT #7: DRINK NO ALCOHOL.

It's been part of the Belly Off! diet plan from day 1. But now we'd like you to follow the no-booze rule for 6 weeks instead of the original 4. Abstaining will dramatically improve your weight-loss results. Why? Reason 1: Because alcohol impairs your body's ability to burn fat by up to 36 percent, according to a Swiss study. Reason 2: Beer, wine, and cocktails are relatively high in empty calories. Reason 3: Drinks often lead to eating a whole school of goldfish-shaped cheese crackers or other salty, high-calorie snack foods. After you've completed your 6-week detox program and workout plan, you can celebrate with a cold one, if you wish. Chances are good that you'll end up limiting your alcohol consumption long after your 6-week detox is over. For hints on sensible social drinking, see "How to Lose Weight at Happy Hour" on page 198.

## POINT #8: EAT MORE FIBER.

Fiber is a weight-loss secret weapon. It reduces the absorption of sugars and fats in your bloodstream, lowers your body's insulin response, and puts the brakes on weight gain by helping you control cravings. Pretty powerful, huh? It's really that important—eating more of it is the best thing you can do to fight diabetes and overweight. Try to increase your fiber to 25 to 30 grams per day.

Admittedly, this is one of the more difficult rules to follow (though it's a lot easier if you're following #4). Most Americans get less than half of the recommended amount of fiber per day because they don't eat the right stuff. (See "Fiber Finder" on the opposite page for a list of foods filled with fiber.) But don't try to go from 0 to 60 overnight. If you try to consume all 30 grams of fiber in that enchilada when your body isn't used to any fiber at all, well, let's just say you had better stay near a toilet and open the windows. Boosting your consumption of fiber should be done gradually so that your body can make a smooth adjustment to digesting the roughage. Introduce high-fiber foods slowly and drink lots of water.

# Fiber Finder

| FOOD | GRAMS OF FIBER |
|---|---|
| COOKED SPLIT PEAS, 1 CUP | 11 |
| NAVY BEANS, 100 GRAMS COOKED | 10.5 |
| PINTO BEANS, 100 GRAMS COOKED | 9 |
| RASPBERRIES, 1 CUP | 8 |
| BLACKBERRIES, 1 CUP | 7.5 |
| CHICKPEAS, 100 GRAMS COOKED | 7.5 |
| WHOLE GRAIN PASTA, 1 CUP COOKED | 6 |
| BRAN FLAKES, ¾ CUP | 5.5 |
| METAMUCIL FIBER WAFERS, 2 | 5 |
| OATS AND OATMEAL, ¾ CUP COOKED | 5 |
| ALMONDS, PEANUTS, OR SUNFLOWER SEEDS, 1 HANDFUL | 4 |
| APPLE, 1 MEDIUM WITH SKIN | 4 |
| WHOLE WHEAT BREAD, 2 SLICES | 4 |
| AIR-POPPED POPCORN, 3 CUPS | 3.5 |
| SPINACH, ½ CUP | 3.5 |
| METAMUCIL POWDERED FIBER SUPPLEMENT, 1 SERVING FOR MIXING IN WATER OR JUICE | 3 |
| RAISINS, 4 TABLESPOONS | 2 |

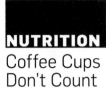

## POINT #9: DRINK LOTS OF WATER.

Water helps fill you up so you don't eat as much, and getting your fill is important for digestion and feeling energized. (And it's a critical teammate of point #7, as an alternative to booze.) Drink at least half of your *current* weight in ounces every day. For example, if you weigh 240 pounds, that's 120 ounces, or fifteen 8-ounce cups. If you weigh 160 pounds, that's ten 8-ounce cups. Remember, we said *at least*. There's nothing wrong with drinking more. For round numbers, anyone would do well to shoot for 12 to 18 cups a day. While that may sound like a lot, it's really not. Most Americans, you included, are walking around dehydrated.

## POINT #10: CONSUME ZERO LIQUID CALORIES FOR THE FIRST WEEK.

This is a tough one—probably the toughest of all of the points on our road map to a flat belly. It means no liquid that has sugar in it. No liquid containing any calories whatsoever. You may drink only water, lemon water, unsweetened tea, or black coffee. No soft drinks (even diet drinks), fruit juices, alcohol, sports drinks, milk, sweetened tea, or coffee. After a week, you may reintroduce a little sugar in your coffee or tea; you can even have a small amount of fruit juice cut with water. But no full-strength juices, sodas, or alcohol for 5 more weeks. This really works. Banish the empty calories!

## POINT #11: AVOID ALL ADDED SUGAR.

Don't use sugar or artificial sweeteners in your coffee and
tea. (This is a must for the first week, but you'll do yourself
a world of good if you can make it a rule for the whole
6 weeks.) Do your best to avoid eating products made with
sugar and artificial sweeteners, such as low-calorie yogurts,
deserts, and baked goods. Avoid jellies and jams, honey,
and brown sugar.

## POINT #12: HUNGRY? THEN YOU SHOULD . . .

Have another apple. Eat more vegetables. Have more of those
foods that are packed with belly-filling water and fiber, yet
are also low in calories. Also, try this: Distract yourself. Studies
show that getting busy with your hands quickly takes your
mind off cravings. Hunger passes fast when you use simple
tricks. Do not allow a grumbling belly to lead your mouth to
a box of doughnuts.

## HOW AM I SUPPOSED TO REMEMBER ALL OF THOSE RULES WHEN I CAN'T EVEN REMEMBER MY WEDDING ANNIVERSARY?

Glad you asked, because here's the answer: The Belly Off!
Detox Points Checklist on page 184. It's a daily reminder to strive
to hit your 12 goals and a confirmation of your success at following
the plan. Make a bunch of copies so you can check off your goals
as you hit them.

# Belly Off! Detox Points Checklist

| | MON | TUES | WED | THURS | FRI | SAT | SUN |
|---|---|---|---|---|---|---|---|
| **1.** I hit my daily calorie goal. | | | | | | | |
| **2.** I ate no fast food. | | | | | | | |
| **3.** I ate a boring lunch. | | | | | | | |
| **4.** Vegetables and fruits were my primary sources of carbs. Beans were my only other source of carbs. | | | | | | | |
| **5.** I ate 1 gram of lean protein per pound of my GOAL body weight. | | | | | | | |
| **6.** I ate 0.25 gram of healthy fat per pound of my GOAL body weight. | | | | | | | |
| **7.** I drank no alcohol. | | | | | | | |
| **8.** I ate ≥ 25 grams of fiber. | | | | | | | |
| **9.** I drank at least half of my CURRENT body weight in ounces of water. | | | | | | | |
| **10.** I drank NO liquid calories. | | | | | | | |
| **11.** I avoided added sugar and didn't eat any artificial sweeteners. | | | | | | | |
| **12.** If I was still hungry, I only snacked on vegetables or fruit. | | | | | | | |

# A DAY ON THE BELLY OFF! DETOX PLAN

Let's look at what this plan might mean for your stomach. Now, what's below is just an example and will change depending on your goal weight, but it will give you a practical frame of reference.

Let's say you are 184 pounds and want to get down to your college weight of 160 pounds. You would multiply your goal weight of 160 by 10 to get 1,600 calories, your daily limit. Below is a sample meal plan that incorporates the detox points above and spreads those 1,600 calories across five meals for the day.

Now you might be saying to yourself, "1,600 calories! I'd starve on that kind of diet!"

Well, no, you really wouldn't "starve." If you examine the sample meal plan below, you'll see that you are getting good quality nutrition. What's being cut out are all those empty calories you were previously eating—the sugary drinks, the snack foods, and other high-glycemic processed carbohydrates. That's why we call it a detox. A low-calorie diet is critical to effective weight loss, so shooting for around 1,600 calories is not an unreasonable goal for anyone. But many of you will have a goal weight greater than 160 pounds. That's fine; simply increase your portion sizes or add a few more side dishes to each meal to increase your calories.

## A SAMPLE 1,600-CALORIE DETOX DAY OF NUTRITION

### BREAKFAST
**400 CALORIES**

- 2 cups of water (with a squeeze of citrus or sliced cucumber, if desired)
- 2 whole eggs cooked with cooking spray, with broccoli and several cups of spinach (or vegetables of your choice)

---

**WEIGHT LOSS**

## 5 Snacks Under 100 Calories

- 2 corn tortillas (6 inches each) and 2 table-spoons of salsa
- 5 fresh apricots
- 4 oz of honey-flavored Greek-style yogurt
- 1 cup of pineapple chunks and 2 teaspoons of shredded coconut
- 24 pistachios

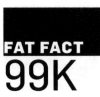

sautéed in 1 teaspoon of olive oil, topped with a slice
of cheese (or a small handful of shredded cheese)

- 1 cup blueberries (or fruit of your choice)

## MORNING SNACK
### 200 CALORIES

- 1 handful of almonds (or nuts of your choice) and 1 apple
(or fruit of your choice)

## LUNCH
### 350 CALORIES

- 2 cups of water (with a squeeze of citrus or sliced cucumber,
if desired)
- Large salad made with a base of 3 to 4 cups of lettuce and
other vegetables (go for a variety of colorful vegetables);
$\frac{1}{2}$ cup of black beans, drained; and 4 oz of grilled chicken
(or tuna, or other source of protein). Mix together with the
juice of 1 squeezed orange and 1 tablespoon of balsamic
vinaigrette dressing.

## AFTERNOON SNACK OR POST-WORKOUT SNACK
### 300 CALORIES

- 2 cups of water (with a squeeze of citrus or sliced cucumber,
if desired)
- Small salad made from 1 small can of salmon; $\frac{1}{2}$ avocado,
sliced; 1 tomato, cut into wedges; a pinch of crushed black
pepper and a pinch of kosher salt. Mix together with
1 teaspoon of balsamic vinaigrette dressing.

# Cut the Fried and the Fast

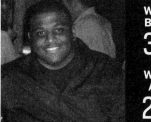

**Weight Before**

# 375

**Weight After**

# 205

# LORENZO TAYLOR

CHICAGO, IL

THE BELLY OFF! CLUB, MARCH 2011

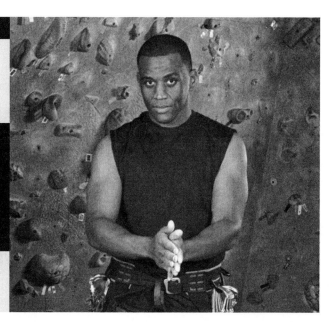

### THE WAKE-UP CALL

I'm a big guy—why fight it? That's what I'd been telling myself since middle school. Deep down, my weight really embarrassed me. College graduation is supposed to be a time of celebration, but I was in a panic: I'd be leaving a comfortable place full of friends who had already accepted me. I'd have to find a job, and I worried that potential employers might see my weight as a liability. Even worse, I was obese and entering the postcollege world of dating. I promised myself on the day of graduation that instead of accepting my "fate," I'd lose the weight.

### HOW I CHANGED

I grew up in the South, where if it wasn't fast food, it was fried food. I lost 15 pounds the first month just by swearing off the junk. I watched my carbs, ate lean proteins, and added vegetables to my meals. I filled up on an omelet for breakfast, a big salad for lunch, and pan-seared chicken with steamed asparagus for dinner, plus I snacked on fruit throughout the day. When I slipped up and ate fast food, I realized that I liked the food I cooked more.

I started running, and that first run was brutal. I doubt I made it 10 minutes. But each time I went out,

I could last longer. Soon I was logging miles instead of minutes. After finishing an 8-K, the sense of accomplishment gave me a huge boost. I added more cardio—like cycling and working out on the elliptical machine. But I was still weak, so I started lifting—doing free-weight exercises, like the bench press—until I could hit my goal of doing bodyweight exercises like dips and pullups. Pretty soon I was building muscle, too.

### THE REWARD

In high school and college, I used to imagine losing weight, walking into a room, and people telling me, "Wow. You look great." Now I hear it from old friends, new co-workers, and my doctor. I can't tell you how good that feels. It pushes me to keep going.

### DINNER
**350 CALORIES**

- 4 oz of grilled chicken (or lean protein of your choice) marinated in balsamic vinaigrette
- 1 grilled red pepper and ½ grilled zucchini (or vegetables of your choice), marinated in balsamic vinaigrette
- 1 small sweet potato, baked

# THE BELLY OFF! 24-HOUR FAST

## HOW IT CAN HELP YOU TAKE YOUR BELLY OFF . . . *FASTER!*

Take a day off . . . from eating, that is. It's not going to kill you. In fact, "very occasional fasting can offer a unique approach to understanding the difference between physiological and psychological hunger," says Dr. Mohr. A daylong fast is an easy, safe, and effective way to get a better grip on hunger and cravings. And it can even help you lose weight.

Everyone eats for reasons other than physical hunger:

- Fear
- Stress
- Boredom
- Fatigue
- Anger
- Elation
- Sadness
- Because the Lakers are playing tonight

Each of these emotional triggers to eating makes it difficult to ultimately understand what it's truly like to be physiologically hungry. The goal of a fasting day is not to cut calories but to recognize the feeling of pure, empty-belly hunger. It may be a feeling you haven't had since you spent an insane day at work without having eaten since dinner the night before. Or maybe since you were an infant crying for milk.

Some new research has shown that fasting on alternating days can help people to drop weight, even when they pig out on their eating days. But the subjects could not maintain their weight loss over time. Alternate-day fasting is tough to sustain.

Some people fast because they believe it can "detox" the body, cleaning it of chemicals and impurities, but there's no evidence that fasting does any of that. You have a much better detox system that works 24/7: your body. It removes toxins efficiently through your liver, colon, kidneys, lungs, and skin (via sweat).

The fast we recommend is purely for the experience and for learning purposes. You'll gain power over food for a day and relearn how your body feels when it needs fuel. By experiencing a fast, you may be more likely to recognize when you are reaching for food out of anxiety, boredom, or other psychological reasons.

Give a 24-hour fast a try. It's simple. Here's the deal: Choose a weekday to fast. (Weekends are much more difficult because you aren't busy at work and you are home and in close proximity to the refrigerator.) Tuesday? Good. After dinner on Monday evening, have nothing more to eat for the rest of the night. Go to sleep. Before you know it, 6 a.m. will arrive and you'll already be halfway through your fast. Keep up with your water drinking, but have no coffee, tea, or juice, and eat no food until 24 hours have passed, which will be around 6 p.m. on Tuesday night. Recognize and write down how your body feels, having been so rudely denied regular feeding. It'll be very different from the feeling that sends you reaching for a candy bar 2 hours after you eat a big lunch. And we believe that you'll find that fasting isn't so hard. You'll feel a few hunger pangs, but they'll soon pass, especially if you keep your mind and body busy with work. You'll learn that you do have willpower and control over your hunger. You'll realize that you didn't shrivel up like a weed in a parched field. You will survive—smarter and stronger in your resolve to combat mindless eating.

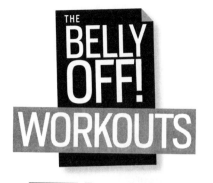

Chapter 8

# THE KEEP-IT-SIMPLE DIET

## Drop Pounds and Fight Flab with This List of the Best Belly Off! Weight-Loss Foods

V ariety is great when you are shopping for a new tie or a pair of shoes for work. Having lots of options is nice when the kids want a trendy crossbreed dog but everyone on the block already has either a yorkiepoo or a goldendoodle. (You go for the schnoodle.)

When it comes to your diet and losing weight, however, variety?

**NUTRITION**
## Eat Naked

Choosing ½ cup of unshelled pistachio nuts instead of ½ cup of candy-coated Peanut M&Ms will save you 90 calories.

Not so good. As we mentioned in the previous chapter, studies show that the more food options humans are faced with, the more food they tend to consume. We're hardwired to take advantage of the bounty of life's all-you-can-eat buffet. And nowhere does that become more problematic for someone trying to take his or her belly off than the grocery store.

Did you know that the average supermarket contains 47,000 different products? Sure, that includes nonedibles like 15 kinds of bathroom tissue and seasonal items like fireworks and plastic reindeer for your lawn. But that still leaves an enormous variety of foodstuffs, including, by our last count, 67 different types of breakfast cereal.

Decisions, decisions. You can blame your belly (in part, at least), on all of those decisions you make at the grocery store. Your willpower, psychologists say, is compromised when you are forced to make a lot of choices. And where do you have to make more choices on a weekly basis than at a grocery store?

A revealing study in the *Journal of Personality and Social Psychology* explored the impact of decision-making on self-control. The experiment involved two groups of students. One group was tasked with choosing between different products in a number of different categories, including T-shirts, scented candles, shampoo brands, socks, and candy. In all, they made about 290 decisions. The no-choice group was asked to write down their opinions of eight advertisements. Both tasks took the same amount of time. Afterward, the groups were given a classic psychological test that measures self-control. Each individual was asked to submerge his or her arm in ice water for as long as he or she could stand the pain. The result: People who were given the decision-making tasks removed their arms from the freezing water much sooner than the people who didn't have to make exhaustive decisions earlier in the day. The researchers say that the same energy that is used for self-control is used for making decisions and that the stress of decision-making depletes the energy required for self-control. Thus, the burned-out decision-makers gave up sooner.

This is why, the researchers say, a dieter who can say no to a jelly doughnut for breakfast cannot, after a day of making tough decisions at work, resist a slice of chocolate cake after dinner. It's also why a grocery shopper who has spent an hour deciding between this box of cereal and that, or between Boston Cream Pie–flavored yogurt and blueberry, can't resist the rack of candy bars at the checkout.

So how do you work around this? Make shopping a no-brainer. Cut down on the decisions you are forced to make by going into that grocery store with a plan: a short list of healthy essentials to form the backbone of your meals. No, it's not exciting. Eating the same foods day after day, week after week is a little boring (unless you get creative and take advantage of the recipes starting on page 210), but it is an extremely effective strategy for weight loss. Stick to a small, core group of foods and you will make it far easier to control the number of calories you consume. You'll get out of the grocery store faster than ever before, too, and without the candy bars.

Here's a list of weight-loss power foods that will build muscle, satisfy your hunger, and improve your health. Use it and the handy grocery checklist at the end of this chapter to simplify your shopping life.

## HEALTH
### Pie Eyed

Researchers at Tufts University found that eating lots of baked goods and other high-glycemic carbohydrates that quickly raise blood sugar can make you nearly 50 percent more likely to suffer from age-related macular degeneration, a leading cause of vision loss. Just another great reason to switch to low-glycemic carbohydrates like those found in legumes, nuts, and whole grains.

# AVOCADOS

Adding chunks of fresh avocado to torn pieces of lettuce is a delicious way to make a salad more substantial and satisfying because avocado is loaded with heart-healthy monounsaturated fat. Many studies have shown that the oleic acid in avocado can improve your cholesterol levels, reduce triglycerides, and improve blood flow to your brain.

# BEANS

Researchers examining results from the National Health and Nutrition Examination Survey report that people who consumed beans were 23 percent less likely to have big bellies than people who said they never ate them.

If you're looking to keep your diet simple, there's no better place to start than beans. Providing protein, fiber, and slow-burning energy, they're the perfect food to stock your pantry with because they can form a nutritious foundation for any meal. You can easily incorporate beans into your diet every day. And you'd be making a huge overhaul to your diet, cheaply. Next to eggs, beans (dried or canned) are the least-expensive sources of protein to be had. It's hard to find a bean that isn't really good for you—except, of course, for jellybeans. Stock these:

- **Black beans.** Great with eggs or packed into a burrito, they are rich in special antioxidant compounds that boost brainpower. Just ½ cup will deliver one-third of your daily fiber needs.

- **Garbanzo beans (aka chickpeas).** Toss them into every salad you make. High in fiber, they quickly stabilize blood sugar, lowering your risk of type 2 diabetes.

- **Kidney beans.** This legume is a top source of thiamine and riboflavin, two B vitamins that strengthen memory and help your body use energy efficiently.

- **Lentils.** Rich in folate, iron, and cholesterol-lowering soluble fiber. Make a big pot of lentil soup. Freeze half, eat some today, and have leftovers for days afterward.

# DATES AND DRIED FIGS

Sugary sweet, they are nature's candy, but unlike Swedish fish, a ½-cup serving will provide about one-quarter of your day's fiber quota. Because the fiber fills you up, they make a nice hunger-stifling snack. And they contain potassium, vitamin $B_6$, and magnesium.

# EGGS

If you're scrambling to find the perfect diet food, it's hard to beat an egg. (Sorry, couldn't resist.)

A study in *Nutrition Research* showed that men who ate eggs for breakfast consumed fewer calories over the course of the next 24 hours than men who had a bagel for breakfast. Even though the morning meal for both groups contained the same number of calories, the egg eaters ended up swallowing 264 fewer calories by the end of the day. Eggs contain more essential amino acids per calorie than any other food. There are nine essential amino acids that cannot be made by the human body, so they must be obtained through food—and eggs contain all of them. The aminos are crucial for protein synthesis, metabolism, and muscle building. In one egg, you get it all—plus about 6 grams of protein and just 72 calories. Eat the yolks; that's where you find most of the nutrients, and recent studies show no connection between eating eggs and increased cholesterol or more heart attacks in healthy people. Choose organic eggs, if possible; they're tastier and richer in nutrients. Or try omega-3 eggs. Hens fed a diet rich in flaxseed produce eggs that are as high in the omega-3 fatty acids EPA and DHA as many species of fish.

**MUSCLE**

## The Secret Behind Popeye's Guns

In a laboratory study, researchers found that treating human muscle cells with a compound found in spinach increased protein synthesis by 20 percent, which would allow muscle tissue to repair itself faster.

# FAT-FREE MILK

One cup delivers 76 milligrams more calcium and many fewer calories than the same amount of whole milk. Milk is an ideal muscle food because the protein in it is about 80 percent casein and 20 percent whey. The former is digested slowly, so it provides your body with a steady stream of muscle-builder, while whey protein is quickly broken down into amino acids and absorbed into your bloodstream, making it a good protein to consume right after a workout. In fact, chocolate milk has been found to be as effective or better than sports drinks at replacing glucose in fatigued muscles; this is due to milk's additional electrolytes and higher fat content.

If you can, buy organic fat-free milk. Studies in the United Kingdom found that organic milk contains higher levels of omega-3s and conjugated linoleic acid, due to all the grass and clover organic cows consume. CLA, by the way, is a fatty acid that can reduce body fat and boost muscle growth.

# FISH

Fish isn't the most convenient or easiest food to prepare, so to get more of this good source of low-calorie protein and omega-3 fatty acids, stock up on canned albacore tuna and sardines packed in olive oil or water for quick lunches and snacks. Sardines are particularly rich in bone-strengthening calcium because you actually eat the soft bones in the tiny fish. When you have more time, visit your fishmonger for fresh salmon. Choose sockeye, the wild Alaskan salmon, because it has more omega-3 fatty acids than farm-raised salmon, which contains more omega-6s due to the grain-infused feed the farmed fish are given. Wild salmon also may be lower in PCBs and dioxins than farm-raised fish is, and you can eliminate many of the contaminants by removing the skin after cooking; that's where most are concentrated. Want more omega-3s? Try grilling a mackerel fillet. One serving contains twice the amount found in salmon.

# FRUIT

Yes, all fruit has sugar in it—fructose. But it also has tons of vitamins, fiber, water, and health benefits that far outweigh the bump to your blood sugar. A strawberry is not a Jolly Rancher. Eat more fruit. Variety here is good, but if we were to pick five to snack on weekly, they would be:

- **Blueberries and blackberries.** The darker the color of the fruit, the more healthful nutrients it contains, and these both boast more antioxidants than almost any other food. One, called pterostilbene, is known for being particularly powerful in helping the liver break down fat.

- **Apples.** Simply because they can be found everywhere year-round and they are full of fiber and cancer-fighting nutrients. Plant sterols inside apples help to lower cholesterol, and they have some amino acids to bolster testosterone and muscle growth. Eating an apple as an appetizer will help your meal fill you up quicker.

- **Bananas.** One of the best sources of vitamin B$_6$, bananas ease stress and depression and help your body metabolize protein. They are also high in potassium, which lowers blood pressure and risk of heart disease. Great for a grab-and-go breakfast with a slather of peanut butter.

- **Grapefruit.** Drinking unsweetened grapefruit juice or eating half of a grapefruit can help you restore your body's resistance to insulin and help you lose weight. In studies of

## HEALTH
### Keep Your Joints Oiled

Eating olive oil may reduce your chances of suffering from rheumatoid arthritis, according to researchers in Greece who say that the oleic acid in olive oil may reduce the inflammation that contributes to arthritis.

obese people at Scripps Clinic in California, subjects who ate grapefruit during each meal for 12 weeks lost an average of nearly 4 pounds more than dieters who had no grapefruit. (Some grapefruit eaters lost more than 10 pounds.) Researchers attribute the weight loss to a flavonoid in grapefruit that makes insulin more effective at transporting sugar to your cells to be used as energy.

## How to Lose Weight at Happy Hour

Abstaining from beer, wine, and chocolate truffle martinis for 6 weeks will open your eyes to how effective teetotaling can be for weight loss. But if drinking alcohol is something you enjoy at social events and you can't see yourself giving it up for good, there are simple ways to dramatically reduce your alcohol consumption after your hiatus is through.

- **Never go hungry.** Have an apple with a slather of natural peanut butter before you head out for a drink. You'll be far less likely to reach for the fried mozzarella sticks or order the nachos grande if you've already had something filling.

- **Send a gift.** Donate the basket of chips to the guys at the far end of the bar. If snacks are right in front of your nose, you'll automatically reach for them. And the salty stuff will make you drink faster and more. Duh! That's why the bartender put it there!

- **Look around.** To avoid reaching into the bowl of beer nuts, just observe for a few minutes the characters who are reaching *their* grubby paws into the same bowl. Now consider that they have done so after using the toilet. (It's okay, they've washed their hands, right? Are you sure?) Not so hungry for those nuts anymore, are you?

- **Order a chaser.** After every beer or cocktail, order a large glass of ice water. It will fill up your belly,

calorie-free, and you'll automatically consume half the number of drinks—or fewer—than you would without the agua advantage.

- **Stay off the bar stool.** Play a game of pool. Standing burns 1.7 times more calories than sitting. And if you play pool or darts instead of sitting close to the bar, you'll slow down your rate of drinking, you'll be active, and you'll refill less frequently than if you were right next to the bartender.

- **Avoid drinks that come with tiny umbrellas.** Tropical rum drinks and cocktails like margaritas and mojitos pack a caloric wallop thanks to the heavy-duty sugar infusion from the sweet mixers. A piña colada, for example, contains about 392 calories, versus around 145 for a beer or 95 for a vodka tonic (80 proof) made with diet tonic.

- **Choose drinks that come with vegetables.** Order a bloody Mary, extra spicy, with double celery and a carrot stick. A 10-ouncer in a highball glass sports about 125 calories, but with it you're getting lycopene and fiber from the tomato juice and low-cal vegetables to munch on. Plus the spice will cause you to sip more slowly and slightly increase your metabolism. Add a jumbo shrimp and you'll get protein, too.

- **Flag yourself 20 minutes before you plan to leave.** Order a large water with lemon for your last round.

# GREEK YOGURT

Most fruit-flavored low-fat yogurts are filled with sugar or high-fructose corn syrup. They are so high in carbs you might as well eat ice cream. A far better choice is Greek yogurt. The process of separating the yogurt from the watery whey removes lactose and other sugars and more than doubles the protein content to 23 grams, with just 9 grams of carbohydrates. It's thicker and creamier and much more filling than regular yogurt, and it still packs lots of calcium and all the probiotic benefits you get from eating live, active cultures. Add blueberries and crushed walnuts to plain Greek yogurt or, if you need something sweeter, swirl in a spoonful of all-fruit spread.

# GREEN TEA

Japanese studies have shown that drinking green tea may promote fat burning. In one study, subjects who consumed the magic ingredient in tea in an amount equivalent to drinking about 5 cups a day for 12 weeks reduced their body fat by about 5 percent. The special substance? A potent catechin called EGCG. Researchers believe that the catechin may boost metabolism. But more important, hundreds of studies have shown that ECGC has the highest level and broadest spectrum of cancer-fighting activity of any antioxidant. Make a pitcher of unsweetened iced green tea to keep in the fridge, and drink it all day long.

# LEAN MEATS

As you know, lean protein is a classic muscle-building macronutrient and, as a hunger-crusher and metabolism-booster, an effective part of a weight-loss plan. In one study, researchers in

**NUTRITION**
A Fish Tale

Guy orders a pizza with anchovies. Disappointed that there are only four of the tiny fishes on the pie, he complains to the waiter, who responds: "Most people don't like anchovies."

**Fact:** Anchovies are one of the densest sources of omega-3 fatty acids, containing twice as much as tuna. And they're so tiny and low on the food chain, they're virtually free of mercury.

Denmark found that men who substituted protein for 20 percent of their carbohydrates were able to boost the number of calories they burned every day by 5 percent.

Beef is an obvious choice because it can be incorporated into so many meals and it's rich in B vitamins that help your body turn food into energy. Focus on lean beef by choosing cuts that have the words *loin* or *round* in their names (like tenderloin or top round steak); these terms indicate a lower concentration of saturated fat. When buying hamburger meat, look for 92 percent lean ground beef. If you can afford organic or grass-fed beef, go for it; you'll avoid the hormones, antibiotics, and pesticides that go into beef cattle on large feedlots. Grass-fed beef is far cleaner and packs double the amount of the antioxidant vitamin E and large doses of omega-3 fats, as well as CLA, the fatty acid that has been shown to encourage weight loss.

To add variety to your meat meals, stock your freezer with other lean proteins like ground turkey breast, chicken, and pork loin.

# NUTS AND SEEDS

Nuts are heart candy. In a study of more than 3,000 African-American men and women, those who ate nuts at least five times a week cut their risk of dying of heart disease by 44 percent compared with people who ate nuts less frequently. Almonds are one of the best to snack on if you're trying to lose weight. One study found that women who ate almonds had higher levels of the hunger-suppressing hormone cholecystokinin in their blood. Choose raw almonds, not the sugar- and salt-coated ones. Snacking on almonds fights hunger pangs thanks to the belly-filling fiber, monounsaturated fat, and protein they contain. For a little variety, try natural almond butter instead of natural peanut butter (both are top-notch for weight control). Other healthful nuts include cashews, which are rich in iron; walnuts, which contain omega-3s and polyphenols that have anti-inflammatory properties; and pistachios, which studies have shown can lower LDL cholesterol by up to 12 percent (based on two servings daily).

Seeds make sense to have on hand. They are nutritional powerhouses that can be easily sprinkled over many foods, especially green salads, to add some satiating fat and a nutty crunch.

- **Flaxseed.** Like all seeds, it has fiber and protein, but it's also one of the top plant sources of a type of omega-3 fatty acid called alpha-linolenic acid (ALA), which supports the cerebral cortex, the area of the brain responsible for processing sensory information.

- **Pumpkin seeds.** Rich in magnesium, a crucial mineral that plays a role in more than 300 bodily functions.

- **Sunflower seeds.** An ounce provides 3 grams of fiber and good doses of the anti-aging nutrients selenium and vitamin E.

**FAT FACT**
# 580
Average number of calories that Americans consume every day in snacks.

# VEGETABLES

Don't overcomplicate the produce section. Anything you grab here is richer in nutrients and a lot better for your waistline and health than anything you'll find boxed or bagged in the middle aisles of the grocery story. But if you're making a list (or using ours), add these power veggies to your cart.

- **Broccoli.** You can't go wrong with this on your plate. Broccoli is an all-star food, a cruciferous vegetable like cauliflower and cabbage, which contains abundant amounts of the powerful phytonutrient compound sulforaphane, which has

## Redeeming the Hot Dog

Nobody would call a frankfurter the healthiest of foods, but there is a way to trim a dog's calories: Don't eat the starchy bun. Instead, wrap your hot-off-the-grill dog in a nutrition-rich leaf of romaine or green leaf lettuce. You'll save virtually empty calories and 19 grams of carbohydrates.

been shown to prevent cancer and remove toxins from cells. Broccoli also has high concentrations of vitamins A, C, and K, plus folate and fiber.

- **Kale.** Sautéed with olive oil and garlic and tossed with cannellini beans, kale is a terrific side dish. Some even enjoy it as a meal in itself. And this often-overlooked green is a veritable multivitamin on a stem, boasting 15 vitamins and minerals, from A to zeaxanthin and K, E, C, and lutein in between. Once you tire of kale, try its cousin, Swiss chard.

- **Spinach.** This should be on your grocery list weekly. Extremely versatile, it can be steamed as a side dish, made the backbone of a garden salad, chopped and tossed into scrambled eggs, or sandwiched between turkey and tomatoes on whole wheat bread. Studies show that spinach boosts protein synthesis, elevating it to muscle-maker status. It's rich in iron, which transports oxygen to your cells. It contains calcium, phosphorus, potassium, zinc, selenium, and vitamin K, and it's one of the best foods for lowering your risk of age-related macular degeneration.

- **Romaine lettuce.** Have these crunchy leaves on hand and you'll end up eating more salads. Low in calories, with a pleasant, light flavor akin to iceberg lettuce, romaine is robust in nutrition comparatively, with lots of beta-carotene, vitamin K, folate, and eight times more vitamin C than iceberg.

- **Bell peppers.** Choose the ripe red, yellow, or orange peppers over the immature greens. The brighter-colored bells contain many more times the antioxidants. For example, a red bell has nearly twice the vitamin C of a green bell and about nine times the vitamin A. The extra time spent

**BELLY OFF! WORKOUTS**

# SHOPPING LIST

___ Apples, bananas, blueberries, grapefruit

___ Avocados

___ Beans and legumes

___ Bell peppers (red, orange)

___ Broccoli and cauliflower

___ Brown rice

___ Cheeses

___ Dates and dried figs

___ Eggs

___ Fat-free milk

___ Fish (fresh, canned)

___ Flaxseed, pumpkin seeds, sunflower seeds

___ Greek yogurt

___ Green tea

___ Lean beef, poultry

___ Nuts and nut butters

___ Oats

___ Quinoa

___ Spinach, kale, Swiss chard, romaine lettuce

___ Whole grain bread

basking in the sun while on the plant also makes them sweeter. Cut-up brightly colored peppers make ideal snacks because their water and fiber content make them very filling and their crunch is as satisfying as a hard pretzel—almost.

# WHOLE GRAINS

The higher fiber content of whole grains makes them a much better choice than white rice, refined cereals, and breads made from wheat flour—plus they can help you reduce belly fat. In a study reported in the *American Journal of Clinical Nutrition*,

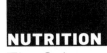

## The Color Guard

Eat a different colored fruit or vegetable at every snack or meal to keep your body stoked with antioxidants. Since many vitamins that protect cells against free radicals are water-soluble, they stay in your body for only 4 to 6 hours and need to be replenished if you're going to keep yourself in optimum disease-fighting shape.

dieters who switched to eating five servings of whole grains every day for 12 weeks lost twice as much belly fat as dieters who ate refined carbohydrates. Here are some good grain foods to stock.

- **Brown rice.** Always substitute brown for white rice. White rice is devoid of fiber, while brown boasts 4 grams a serving, plus more minerals and protein.

- **Oats.** You have a few choices for this hot breakfast meal: rolled oats in two styles, instant and old-fashioned, and steel-cut oats. As the name suggests, instant oatmeal is the quickest to cook—just add boiling water. Old-fashioned oatmeal (or "groats") takes 5 minutes to cook. Both offer good protection against heart disease and type 2 diabetes, as long as you stay away from the "flavored" oats that are loaded with sugar. (It's better to choose the plain variety and sweeten it with fruit.) But your best choice is steel-cut oats. Because they aren't rolled, they take half an hour to cook. And in your gastrointestinal tract, the unrolled oats take longer to digest, which results in a slower release of glucose into your bloodstream. That makes steel-cut oats a top-notch breakfast for people with prediabetes.

- **Quinoa.** Pronounced KEEN-wah, this nutty-tasting South American grain delivers about twice the protein of brown rice, and that protein consists of branched-chain and essential amino acids, just like the ones contained in eggs. This is a grain that builds muscle. It contains some healthy fats and it's a good deal lower in carbs than other grains. It even tastes great for breakfast and cooks up like rice in about 15 minutes.

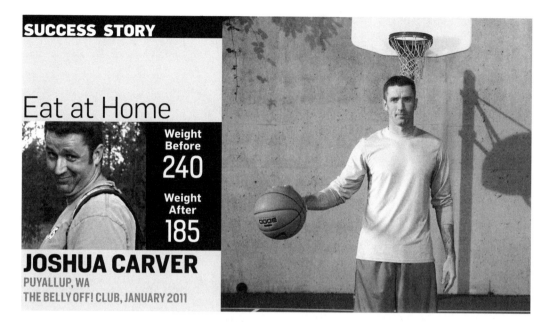

## SUCCESS STORY

# Eat at Home

**Weight Before**
## 240

**Weight After**
## 185

# JOSHUA CARVER
**PUYALLUP, WA**
**THE BELLY OFF! CLUB, JANUARY 2011**

**THE WAKE-UP CALL**

In my job as a pharmaceutical salesman, my gut really started growing. Man, it was embarrassing: There I was, a clearly unhealthy guy talking to health-care providers about drugs that lower cholesterol and treat diabetes. How could I be taken seriously? Then I blew out my knee and ankle. Shortly after the operation to repair them, I had to prepare for my son's baptism—and I needed a new suit. I stood in the fitting room, barely squeezing into a pair of size 38 pants, and thought about how much my weight was costing me. I needed to change.

**HOW I CHANGED**

When you work long hours, as I do, you assume that fast food is your only dinner option. But I realized I could cook a meal at home in the same amount of time it took me to drive to a fast-food restaurant. I didn't need to be a great cook—healthy meals are simple to make. Breakfast is a few eggs with turkey, rolled into a wrap. Lunch is a grilled chicken sandwich or salad. Dinner is a lean protein, like shrimp or salmon, with a side of steamed broccoli or green beans. All good stuff.

I started hitting the gym after work—both to de-stress and, at first, to lift when fewer people were watching. I started slow and gradually added weight. I'd walk at least a mile every weekday on my lunch break. On weekends, I'd run 3 or 4 miles. I skipped the cart during golf, and I coached my 9-year-old's baseball team. I made fitness fun.

**THE REWARD**

After I lost the weight, I felt better representing my company. My sales improved. I called in sick less. My bosses even asked me to talk with the rest of my team about living a healthy lifestyle. Now I think of myself as a whole new person.

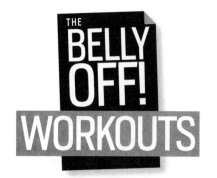

Chapter 9

# THE NEW BELLY OFF! DIET RECIPES

## Great–Tasting, Flab–Fighting Meals to Fuel Your Belly Off! Workouts

The most effective fat-burning machines on earth cannot be found in any gym or health club, because they're right inside your kitchen. You can't miss them! They are large and heavy, and one is probably stained with last night's spaghetti sauce. With daily use, both your refrigerator and cooking range can help you lose weight and shape up quicker and easier than any high-tech weight-stack machine or iPod-enabled treadmill.

A recent analysis of dozens of food consumption studies from around the world reported in the journal *Obesity Reviews* revealed something very interesting about the power of do-it-yourself food. Overwhelmingly, when people cooked and ate at home, they ate healthier food, and when people ate meals outside the home, on average they consumed more calories, fat, and sodium and less vitamin C, vitamin A, calcium, and fiber. In the United States, the review showed, men consume 25 percent of their daily energy outside of the home, compared with 15 percent for women. Other studies show that when people eat just *one* fast-food meal, on average, they consume 500 more calories than they would if they prepared and ate that meal at home.

You don't have to bench press your fridge to get fit—just fill it with the healthy ingredients for a homemade meal. Cooking at home puts *you* in control of your food, not some fast-food conglomerate or spatula-wielding SpongeBob in a paper hat. By not ordering off a menu, you cut out the thousands of food choices that tempt you to overeat. You automatically reduce your consumption of unhealthy artificial additives typically found in processed foods—additives that can lead to weight gain. By actually handling the food you'll eventually swallow, you instinctively eat fresher, more-healthful fare.

This chapter is filled with delicious recipes to make mealtimes exciting. These recipes were selected because they are heavy on nutrients but light on carb and calorie density. We've put our focus on the most challenging meals of the day— breakfast and dinner—because that's when you are more likely to cook something. For a workday lunch, brown-bag a turkey or egg salad sandwich or leftovers from dinner, or have a salad with some protein on top. Keep it simple.

## SUCCESS STORY

# Cook Once, Eat for a Week

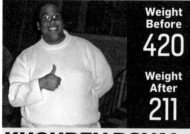

**Weight Before**
## 420

**Weight After**
## 211

# KHOUREY ROYAL

**CHARLOTTESVILLE, VA**
**THE BELLY OFF! CLUB, APRIL 2010**

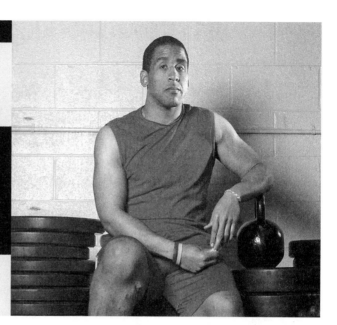

**THE WAKE-UP CALL**
I grew up a chubby kid, with a dad who was bedridden with weight-related heart problems. I vowed not to end up like my father.

**HOW I CHANGED**
I have a good friend who introduced me to weights, and it changed my life. Now my typical week's program includes lunges, box jumps, and step-ups for my lower body, along with curls, dumbbell kickbacks, and bench presses for my upper body.
I make sure my meals include lean meats, fruits or vegetables, and whole grains. That takes planning. So I make a big batch of food on the weekend and eat well all week long. (See Royal's recipe for a big batch of jerk chicken, below.)

**THE REWARD**
I've changed my body. I have a bigger chest, smaller waist, defined arms, and trimmer legs, but I'm not satisfied yet. I'm having too much fun in the gym. Now I'm looking for more muscle definition. New challenges keep me hungry.

## Royal's Jerk Chicken

Royal uses chicken thighs for their extra flavor and works the rub under the skin to help infuse the meat with the spices.

- ¼ cup white wine vinegar
- 1 tablespoon minced fresh ginger
- 4 cloves garlic, minced
- 2 jalapeño peppers, minced
- 1½ tablespoons light brown sugar
- 1½ tablespoons vegetable oil
- 1 tablespoon ground allspice
- 1½ teaspoons kosher salt
- 2 pounds skin-on, bone-in chicken thighs

In a medium bowl, combine the vinegar, ginger, cloves, jalapeños, sugar, oil, allspice, and salt. Then dump the spice rub and the chicken into a zipper-lock bag, shake to coat, and refrigerate for 1 hour.

Remove the chicken from the bag, and discard the marinade. Heat a grill pan over medium heat and grill the chicken until it's cooked through, 10 to 15 minutes on each side. Serve it with brown rice, grilled vegetables, or a mixed-greens salad with sliced avocado and mango.

# BELLY OFF! BREAKFASTS

## The Sicilian
(spinach and tomato omelet)

|       |                                                      |
|-------|------------------------------------------------------|
| 3     | egg whites                                           |
| 1     | egg                                                  |
| 1/4   | teaspoon dried oregano                               |
| 1/4   | teaspoon dried basil                                 |
|       | Pinch of garlic salt                                 |
|       | Pinch of black pepper                                |
| 1     | cup baby spinach                                     |
| 1/2   | fresh plum or Roma tomato, seeded and finely chopped |
| 2     | slices low-sodium deli ham (1 ounce each)            |
| 1/4   | cup marinara sauce                                   |
| 1     | tablespoon ricotta cheese                            |
| 1/4   | cup shredded mozzarella cheese                       |

**1.** In a small bowl, whisk together the egg whites, egg, oregano, basil, garlic salt, and pepper until well blended. Set aside.

**2.** Coat a small omelet pan or skillet with cooking spray. Heat over medium heat. Add the spinach, tomato, and ham, and cook for 3 minutes, stirring, until the spinach is wilted. Remove to a bowl.

**3.** Coat the pan again with the cooking spray. Pour in the egg mixture and occasionally lift the edges of the cooked egg to allow uncooked egg to run underneath.

**4.** In a microwaveable bowl, stir together the marinara and ricotta. Cover with a paper towel and microwave for 30 seconds, or until hot.

**5.** Once the egg is cooked on the top, put the spinach mixture on half of the omelet and sprinkle with the mozzarella cheese. Flip the plain half of the omelet over the filling and cover and cook for 2 minutes, or until the cheese melts.

**6.** Put the omelet on a plate. Pour the marinara mixture over the top.

MAKES 1 SERVING.

**Per serving:** 314 calories, 39 g protein, 17 g carbohydrates, 10 g fat (4 g saturated), 3 g fiber, 1,331 mg sodium

## Hill O' Beans Hotcakes
(high-fiber pancakes)

| | |
|---|---|
| 1 | cup canned navy beans, rinsed and drained |
| 2 | teaspoons canola oil |
| 2 | tablespoons honey |
| 2 | teaspoons vanilla extract |
| $\frac{1}{4}$ | teaspoon salt |
| $1\frac{1}{3}$ | cups rolled oats |
| $\frac{1}{2}$ | cup whipped cream |
| 1 | cup blueberries or sliced strawberries |

**1.** Place the beans, oil, honey, vanilla, salt, and 1 cup of water in a blender. Blend for 2 minutes. Add the oats and blend for 1 additional minute, or until pureed and well blended.

**2.** Coat a large nonstick skillet or griddle with cooking spray. Heat over medium heat. Drop the batter $\frac{1}{4}$ cup at a time onto the skillet and cook for 4 minutes, or until the edges start to look dry. Flip the pancakes and cook for 3 minutes or until browned on both sides.

**3.** Divide between 2 plates. Top with the whipped cream and berries.

MAKES 2 SERVINGS.

**Per serving:** 624 calories, 20 g protein, 92 g carbohydrates, 20 g fat (7 g saturated), 14 g fiber, 891 mg sodium

## Omega Toast
(French toast with flaxseed)

2  egg whites

¼  cup fat-free milk

1  scoop vanilla whey protein powder

1  tablespoon ground flaxseed

3  slices whole wheat bread

1½  cups sliced bananas or strawberries

6  tablespoons real maple syrup

**1.** Combine the egg whites, milk, protein powder, and flaxseed in a shallow bowl. Whisk to blend, and then pour the mixture into a baking dish.

**2.** Dip all 3 pieces of the bread in the egg mixture. Let them stand for 2 minutes, turning once, or until they absorb all of the egg mixture. If the bread is dense, stab it a few times with a fork.

**3.** Coat a nonstick skillet with cooking spray. Heat the skillet over medium heat. Add the bread slices and cook for 4 minutes, turning once or until browned.

**4.** Serve each slice of toast with ½ cup of the fruit and 2 tablespoons of the syrup. (If you're planning to treat yourself to this during your detox, the fruit will provide enough sweetness to help you eliminate the syrup.)

MAKES 3 SERVINGS.

**Per serving:** 250 calories, 14 g protein, 44 g carbohydrates, 3 g fat (2 g saturated), 5 g fiber, 283 mg sodium

# Cheeseberry Bluecakes
(blueberry pancakes with extra protein)

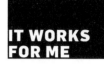

| | |
|---|---|
| ¼ | cup water |
| 2 | tablespoons sugar |
| 1 | cup blueberries |
| ¼ | cup all-purpose flour |
| ⅓ | cup reduced-fat ricotta cheese |
| 2 | eggs |
| 2 | slices Canadian bacon |

**1.** Place the water and sugar in a small saucepan over medium heat. Add ¾ cup of the blueberries and simmer to dissolve the sugar and thicken the sauce, about 2 minutes. Set the sauce aside.

**2.** Mix the flour, ricotta, and eggs together. Add the remaining ¼ cup of blueberries to the batter. Heat a nonstick skillet over medium heat. Add the Canadian bacon slices and cook for about a minute. Remove from the pan and set aside.

**3.** Coat the same skillet with olive oil spray. Drop spoonfuls of the batter onto the hot skillet to form pancakes. Cook for 2 minutes. Turn and cook for 1 additional minute. Remove and serve with the bacon. Top the pancakes with the blueberry sauce.

MAKES 2 SERVINGS.

**Per serving:** 303 calories, 17 g protein, 38 g carbohydrates, 9 g fat (3 g saturated), 2 g fiber, 472 mg sodium

"I was always a mass-consumption kind of guy, so I had to find healthier ways to fill up. Fiber was the key: Now I always eat oatmeal in the morning, and I snack on a Fiber One bar and a tall glass of water during the day. Another snack I like is popcorn with a little sea salt, cayenne, and Old Bay seasoning. I was never big on fruits, but I enjoy them in a meal-replacement smoothie once or twice a day. My favorite: frozen blueberry and pineapple with a little agave nectar and a base of almond milk."

—Bryn Davis
**Weight Before:**
236 pounds
**Weight After:**
174 pounds
The Belly Off! Club,
September 2010

## The Muffin Man
(blueberry-cinnamon breakfast muffins)

| | |
|---|---|
| 1¼ | cups whole grain pastry or white whole wheat flour |
| ½ | cup old-fashioned rolled oats |
| 2 | teaspoons baking powder |
| 1 | teaspoon baking soda |
| 1 | teaspoon cinnamon |
| ½ | teaspoon salt |
| ⅔ | cup honey |
| ½ | cup fat-free plain yogurt |
| ½ | cup liquid egg whites |
| 1 | cup blueberries |

**1.** Preheat the oven to 350°F. Coat a 12-cup muffin pan with cooking spray, or use paper liners.

**2.** Combine the flour, oats, baking powder, baking soda, cinnamon, and salt in a large bowl. Whisk to blend. Add the honey, yogurt, and egg whites. Stir just until blended. Stir in the blueberries.

**3.** Spoon the batter into the muffin cups, almost filling them. Bake for 20 to 25 minutes. Test for doneness by sticking a toothpick into the middle of a few muffins; if the toothpick is clean (or just has some crumbs on it), they're ready.

**4.** Cool in the pan for 5 minutes. Remove to a rack to cool completely.

MAKES 12 MUFFINS.

**Per serving:** 123 calories, 3 g protein, 28 g carbohydrates, 0.5 g fat (0 g saturated), 2 g fiber, 316 mg sodium

# Let 'Em Eat Cake
(walnut banana bread)

|   |   |
|---|---|
| 3 | medium bananas, smashed |
| 2 | eggs |
| $\frac{1}{2}$ | cup fat-free plain yogurt |
| 1 | teaspoon vanilla extract |
| 2 | cups whole grain pastry or white whole wheat flour |
| $\frac{2}{3}$ | cup packed brown sugar |
| 1 | tablespoon ground flaxseed |
| 1 | teaspoon baking powder |
| 1 | teaspoon baking soda |
| 1 | teaspoon ground cinnamon |
| $\frac{1}{2}$ | teaspoon salt |
| $\frac{1}{2}$ | cup chopped walnuts |
| $\frac{1}{2}$ | cup raisins |

**1.** Preheat the oven to 350°F. Coat a 9 x 5-inch loaf pan with cooking spray.

**2.** Combine the bananas, eggs, yogurt, and vanilla in a medium bowl, and stir to blend.

**3.** Combine the flour, sugar, flaxseed, baking powder, baking soda, cinnamon, and salt in a large bowl. Stir to blend. Stir in the banana mixture just until blended. Stir in the walnuts and raisins.

**4.** Pour the mixture into the loaf pan. Bake for 45 minutes. Stick a toothpick into the middle of the loaf in a few places; if the toothpick is clean (or just has some crumbs on it), the bread is ready. If not, bake for another 3 minutes and recheck. Cool in the pan for 10 minutes. Remove from the pan and cool on a rack.

MAKES 10 SERVINGS.

**Per serving:** 240 calories, 6 g protein, 45 g carbohydrates, 6 g fat (1 g saturated), 4 g fiber, 323 mg sodium

## Lasagna for Breakfast
(egg strata)

1    jar (16 ounces) salsa

4    whole wheat tortillas (8 inches in diameter)

1    teaspoon extra virgin olive oil

½    green bell pepper

3    eggs, beaten

1    tablespoon chopped cilantro

½    cup shredded, reduced-fat Cheddar or Colby cheese

**1.** Preheat the oven to 350°F. Coat a 10 x 8-inch baking dish with cooking spray. Spread 1 cup of the salsa in the pan. Put 2 of the tortillas over the salsa, overlapping them slightly.

**2.** Heat the oil in a skillet over medium heat. Sauté the pepper, stirring, for 3 minutes or until tender-crisp. Stir in the eggs and scramble until almost cooked. Spread over the tortillas in the dish. Sprinkle the cilantro over the eggs.

**3.** Top with the remaining 2 tortillas. Pour the rest of the salsa over the tortillas. Top with the cheese. Bake for 10 to 15 minutes or until the cheese is melted and the strata is hot.

MAKES 2 SERVINGS.

**Per serving:** 519 calories, 26 g protein, 57 g carbohydrates, 20 g fat (8 g saturated), 7 g fiber, 1,570 mg sodium

## It's Beta with Feta
(vegetable-feta omelet)

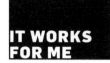

| | |
|---|---|
| 3 | eggs |
| 1 | tablespoon fat-free milk |
| | Pinch of garlic powder |
| 1 | tablespoon olive oil |
| 1/2 | small onion, chopped |
| 1/2 | cup sliced mushrooms |
| 1 | cup baby spinach |
| 1 | tablespoon crumbled reduced-fat feta |
| | Pinch of seasoned pepper |
| 1 | tomato, seeded and chopped |

**1.** Whisk together the eggs, milk, and garlic powder until well blended. Set aside.

**2.** Heat the oil in a small nonstick omelet pan or skillet over medium heat. Add the onion and mushrooms and cook for 4 minutes, stirring, until lightly browned. Remove to a bowl.

**3.** Coat the same pan with the cooking spray. Pour in the egg mixture and occasionally lift the edges of the cooked egg to allow uncooked egg to run underneath.

**4.** Once the egg has set, place the spinach, onion mixture, and feta on half of the omelet. Flip the plain half of the omelet over the filling and cover and cook for 2 minutes, or until the cheese melts.

**5.** Put the omelet on a plate. Top with the tomato.

MAKES 1 SERVING.

**Per serving:** 412 calories, 24 g protein, 14 g carbohydrates, 30 g fat (7 g saturated), 4 g fiber, 382 mg sodium

"For many years, my morning ritual was to stop for a caffe latte on the drive to work. Then my sister pointed out to me that there is a lot of whole milk in it, plus all the calories from the sugar I added. So I switched to regular coffee and gradually cut down on the amount of cream and sugar until my morning ritual was black coffee. Now all I drink is Americano style, black. It saves me about 205 calories a day."

—Scott Bartkowski;
**Weight Before:**
205 pounds
**Weight After:**
184 pounds
The Belly Off! Club
Online, 2010

## The Morning Monster
(open-face egg sandwich)

| | |
|---|---|
| 2 | eggs |
| 1 | tablespoon fat-free milk |
| 1/8 | teaspoon salt |
| 1/8 | teaspoon freshly ground black pepper |
| 2 | teaspoons olive oil |
| 2 | tablespoons shredded Parmesan |
| 3 | slices shaved deli ham (1.5 ounces total) |
| 1 | slice whole wheat or 12 grain bread, toasted |

**1.** Whisk together the eggs, milk, salt, and pepper until well blended. Set aside.

**2.** Heat the oil in a small nonstick omelet pan or skillet over medium heat. Pour in the egg mixture and occasionally lift the edges of the cooked egg to allow uncooked egg to run underneath.

**3.** Sprinkle the Parmesan over half of the omelet. Flip the plain half of the omelet over the filling. Cover and cook for 1 minute or until the cheese melts.

**4.** Put the ham on the toast. Top with the omelet.

MAKES 1 SERVING.

**Per serving:** 395 calories, 29 g protein, 15 g carbohydrates, 25 g fat (7 g saturated), 2 g fiber, 1,245 mg sodium

## Squashed Latkes
(zucchini fritters)

$1\frac{1}{2}$  cups grated zucchini or yellow squash

2  tablespoons grated onion

$\frac{1}{4}$  cup Parmesan cheese

$\frac{1}{4}$  cup whole wheat flour

2  whole eggs, beaten

3  tablespoons plain Greek yogurt

1  tablespoon red pepper flakes (optional)

Sour cream (optional)

**1.** Squeeze the water out of the grated squash. (There will be more than you expect.)

**2.** Combine the zucchini, onion, cheese, flour, eggs, yogurt, and red pepper flakes (if using) in a large bowl. Stir until combined.

**3.** Oil a frying pan with olive oil and drop dollops of the fritter batter into the pan using a large soup spoon. Flatten the zucchini mixture into circles and fry as you would potato pancakes, until both sides are crispy. Garnish with sour cream, if using.

MAKES 2 SERVINGS.

**Per serving:** 213 calories, 15 g protein, 16 g carbohydrates, 11 g fat (5 g saturated), 3 g fiber, 238 mg sodium

## BREAKFAST THAT'S FASTER
## Five morning meals made in a flash

**1.** A slice of sprouted grain bread with 1 tablespoon of almond butter

**2.** A whole wheat tortilla with one slice each of deli turkey breast and cheese, rolled up

**3.** Two microwaveable vegetable-protein sausages on a hot dog roll, topped with organic, low-sugar ketchup

**4.** Vanilla yogurt ($\frac{1}{2}$ cup) topped with a handful of All-Bran Extra Fiber cereal and fresh blueberries

**5.** One scoop of vanilla whey protein mixed into vanilla-flavored organic low-fat milk

## PB & BO
(peanut butter and blueberry oatmeal)

| | |
|---|---|
| ¾ | cup old-fashioned oats |
| ⅛ | teaspoon ground cinnamon |
| ⅛ | teaspoon ground ginger |
| | Pinch of ground cloves |
| | Pinch of salt |
| 1¼ | cups fat-free milk or water |
| ½ | teaspoon vanilla extract |
| ½ | cup fresh or frozen blueberries |
| 1 | tablespoon protein powder |
| 1 | tablespoon peanut butter (natural, if possible) |

**1.** Combine the oats, cinnamon, ginger, cloves, and salt in a microwaveable bowl. Add the milk or water and vanilla, and stir just to combine.

**2.** Microwave on high for 1 minute, stirring once. Remove the bowl from the microwave and stir in the blueberries and protein powder.

**3.** Microwave on high for another 1 to 2 minutes or until thickened, stirring halfway through. Top with the peanut butter.

MAKES 1 SERVING.

**Per serving:** 524 calories, 28 g protein, 73 g carbohydrates, 13 g fat (1 g saturated), 11 g fiber, 335 mg sodium

## Almond Hammer Smoothie

6   ounces almond milk

1   tablespoon almond butter

1   scoop chocolate whey protein powder

½   banana

1   teaspoon ground flaxseed

Combine the almond milk, almond butter, protein powder, banana, flaxseed, and 5 ice cubes in a blender. Blend until smooth, but avoid overblending, which can make the drink too thick and frothy.

MAKES 1 SERVING.

**Per serving:** 299 calories, 24 g protein, 25 g carbohydrates, 13 g fat (1 g saturated), 3 g fiber, 206 mg sodium

## The Dippie Hippie Smoothie

1   cup skim milk

1   scoop chocolate whey protein powder

2   tablespoons nonfat French vanilla creamer

¼   cup low-fat granola

½   frozen banana

1   tablespoon natural peanut butter

2   tablespoons sugar-free hot cocoa mix

Combine the milk, protein powder, creamer, granola, banana, peanut butter, and chocolate mix in a blender. Blend until smooth, but avoid overblending, which can make the drink too thick and frothy.

MAKES 1 SERVING.

**Per serving:** 537 calories, 35 g protein, 77 g carbohydrates, 11 g fat (2 g saturated), 5 g fiber, 242 mg sodium

**WEIGHT LOSS**

## In Thickness and Health

A thicker drink can make you thinner. Researchers at Purdue University found that people stayed full longer when they drank thick drinks than when they drank thin ones, even when the amount of liquid and the calories the drinks contained were equal. The thicker drinks were more effective at stifling hunger longer.

### Coconut Crème Pie Smoothie

8   ounces pineapple juice

1   scoop vanilla whey protein powder

$\frac{1}{2}$   teaspoon coconut extract

1   ounce sweetened or flaked coconut (about $\frac{1}{3}$ cup)

Combine the juice, protein powder, coconut extract, coconut, and 3 ice cubes in a blender. Blend until smooth, but avoid overblending, which can make the drink too thick and frothy.

MAKES 1 SERVING.

**Per serving:** 361 calories, 21 g protein, 45 g carbohydrates, 11 g fat (9 g saturated), 3 g fiber, 124 mg sodium

### Orangemen Smoothie

1   cup skim milk

1   scoop vanilla whey protein powder

2   tablespoons nonfat French vanilla creamer

2   teaspoons frozen orange juice concentrate

1   teaspoon vanilla extract

$\frac{1}{2}$   ripe banana

Combine the milk, protein powder, creamer, juice concentrate, vanilla extract, banana, and 3 ice cubes in a blender. Blend until smooth, but avoid overblending, which can make the drink too thick and frothy.

MAKES 1 SERVING.

**Per serving:** 340 calories, 28 g protein, 49 g carbohydrates, 1 g fat (0 g saturated), 2 g fiber, 172 mg sodium

# BELLY OFF! DINNERS AND SIDES

## Chicken in a Blanket
(Asian chicken and lettuce wraps)

|     |     |
| --- | --- |
| 1 | pound lean ground chicken |
| 4 | scallions, chopped |
| 2 | large carrots, shredded |
| $1\frac{1}{2}$ | teaspoons grated fresh ginger |
| $\frac{1}{8}$ | teaspoon crushed red pepper flakes |
| 2 | tablespoons hoisin sauce |
| 2 | teaspoons rice wine vinegar |
| 2 | cups fresh spinach, chopped |
| 1 | head butterhead lettuce, leaves separated (about 20 large leaves) |
| $\frac{1}{2}$ | cup cilantro leaves |
| $\frac{1}{2}$ | cup mint leaves |
|   | Lime wedges |

**1.** Cook the chicken in a large nonstick skillet set over medium-high heat for 5 minutes, stirring occasionally and breaking up the meat with a spoon.

**2.** Stir in the scallions, carrots, ginger, and crushed red pepper flakes. Cook for 2 minutes more or until the vegetables are tender-crisp and the chicken is no longer pink. Remove from the heat and stir in the hoisin and vinegar. Stir in the spinach until the mixture is well combined.

**3.** To assemble the wraps, spoon about 3 tablespoons of the chicken mixture into a lettuce leaf. Divide the cilantro and mint leaves and place on top of each chicken mixture. Add a drizzle of lime juice and roll the leaf up into a wrap.

MAKES 4 SERVINGS (ABOUT 1 CUP CHICKEN MIXTURE PER SERVING).

**Per serving:** 156 calories, 27 g protein, 11 g carbohydrates, 1 g fat (0 g saturated), 3 g fiber, 250 mg sodium

# Ha-Van-A Side Dish
(Cuban fried rice)

| | |
|---|---|
| 1 | teaspoon olive oil |
| 1 | red bell pepper, chopped |
| 1 | green bell pepper, chopped |
| 1 | cup chopped pineapple |
| 4 | scallions, sliced |
| 1 | large carrot, shredded |
| $\frac{1}{2}$ | small jalapeño pepper, seeded and chopped |
| $1\frac{1}{4}$ | teaspoons dried oregano, crumbled |
| $\frac{3}{4}$ | teaspoon thyme |
| $\frac{1}{4}$ | teaspoon salt |
| 2 | cups cooked brown rice |
| 1 | cup canned black beans, rinsed and drained |
| $\frac{1}{2}$ | pound cooked roast pork, cut into $\frac{3}{8}$-inch pieces (2 cups) |
| $\frac{1}{3}$ | cup fresh orange juice |
| | Lime wedges |

**1.** Heat the oil in a large nonstick skillet over medium-high heat. Add the red and green bell peppers and cook for 5 minutes, stirring occasionally. Stir in the pineapple, scallions, carrot, jalapeño, oregano, thyme, and salt. Stir-fry for 2 minutes.

**2.** Stir in the rice and black beans. Stir-fry for 1 minute. Stir in the pork and orange juice. Stir-fry for 1 minute or until heated through. Serve with lime wedges.

MAKES 4 SERVINGS ($1\frac{1}{2}$ CUPS PER SERVING).

**Per serving:** 373 calories, 23 g protein, 45 g carbohydrates, 11 g fat (4 g saturated), 7 g fiber, 394 mg sodium

# Greens Beans
(sautéed kale and white beans)

2   teaspoons extra virgin olive oil, plus additional for drizzling

1   large clove garlic, minced

1   large head kale, chopped (about 13 cups)

1   can (15 ounces) navy beans, rinsed and drained

$\frac{1}{8}$   teaspoon sea salt

$\frac{1}{8}$   teaspoon cracked black pepper

**1.** Heat the oil in a large skillet over medium heat. Add the garlic and cook for 2 minutes. Add the kale and sauté until wilted, about 4 minutes.

**2.** Add the beans and heat through. Season with the salt and pepper. Drizzle with extra oil.

MAKES 6 SERVINGS.

**Per serving:** 141 calories, 8 g protein, 24 g carbohydrates, 3 g fat (0 g saturated), 5 g fiber, 323 mg sodium

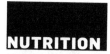

## NUTRITION
## Broaden Your Spreads

Instead of mayonnaise on that sandwich, try a spread of mashed ripe avocado or hummus. Avocados are rich in heart-healthy monounsaturated fat and hummus is made from chickpeas, a good source of fiber and protein.

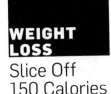

## Slice Off 150 Calories

Make your next sandwich open-faced. By doing without one slice of bread, you'll save that many carb calories.

## It's Greek to Me
### (Mediterranean chicken burgers)

The addition of spinach not only adds nutrients, but also helps to keep these burgers moist and juicy.

| | |
|---|---|
| 4 | scallions, chopped |
| 1 | pound lean ground chicken |
| 2 | cups frozen, dry-packed, leaf spinach, thawed, squeezed dry, and chopped |
| ¼ | cup plain, dried bread crumbs |
| 2 | tablespoons chopped kalamata olives (about 8) |
| ½ | teaspoon dried oregano, crumbled |
| ¼ | teaspoon dried dill |
| | Salt |
| | Freshly ground black pepper |
| 4 | light whole wheat hamburger rolls, split |
| 2 | tomatoes, thinly sliced |
| 1 | cucumber, thinly sliced |
| ¾ | cup plain, low-fat yogurt |

**1.** Preheat an outdoor grill or grill pan over medium heat. Set aside 3 tablespoons of the chopped scallions for the salad. In a large bowl, stir together the chicken, spinach, bread crumbs, olives, oregano, dill, ¼ teaspoon of salt, ¼ teaspoon of black pepper, and the remaining scallions until combined. Shape the mixture into 4 patties, each about 4 inches in diameter.

**2.** Grill the burgers over medium heat for 10 to 12 minutes, or until no longer pink, turning once. Grill the rolls, cut sides down, for 1 minute. Place the burgers on the rolls.

**3.** Arrange the tomato and cucumber slices on a serving plate. In a medium bowl, stir together the yogurt and the remaining 3 tablespoons of scallions. Serve with the salad and burgers.

MAKES 4 SERVINGS.

**Per serving:** 332 calories, 37 g protein, 40 g carbohydrates, 5 g fat (1 g saturated), 10 g fiber, 817 mg sodium

# Crabby Patties
(lump crab cakes)

|       |                                    |
|-------|------------------------------------|
| 8     | ounces lump crabmeat               |
| 1     | large egg                          |
| 1½    | cups panko bread crumbs            |
|       | Freshly ground black pepper        |
| ½     | cup light mayonnaise               |
| 2     | shallots, finely chopped           |
| 2     | tablespoons lemon juice            |
| 2     | tablespoons chopped fresh chives   |
| 2     | tablespoons fresh tarragon         |

**1.** In a large bowl, combine the crabmeat, egg, ¼ teaspoon of black pepper, ½ cup of the panko, ¼ cup of the mayonnaise, half of the shallots, and 1 tablespoon of the lemon juice. Form the mixture into 4 patties. Coat in the remaining bread crumbs.

**2.** In a smaller bowl, combine ⅛ teaspoon of black pepper, the chives, the tarragon, the remaining ¼ cup of mayo, the remaining shallots, and the remaining 1 tablespoon of lemon juice to make the sauce.

**3.** Coat a nonstick skillet with cooking spray and place it over medium heat. Brown the patties in the pan for 4 minutes per side. Top with the sauce and serve.

MAKES 4 SERVINGS.

**Per serving:** 275 calories, 17 g protein, 24 g carbohydrates, 12 g fat (0 g saturated), 1 g fiber, 482 mg sodium

## Noth Shaw Chowda
### (codfish and shrimp tomato chowder)

Make this hearty Gloucester, Massachusetts–inspired seafood soup into a dinner by serving it with a salad of crisp greens and baby spinach topped with diced cucumber and red bell pepper.

| | |
|---|---|
| 1 | teaspoon olive oil |
| 2 | stalks celery, chopped |
| 1 | onion, chopped |
| 1 | can (28 ounces) crushed tomatoes |
| 1 | cup low-sodium chicken broth |
| 2 | small zucchini or summer squash (10 ounces), chopped |
| 1 | green bell pepper, chopped |
| 1 | clove garlic, chopped |
| 1¼ | teaspoons dried oregano |
| ¼ | teaspoon crushed red pepper flakes |
| ¾ | cup no-salt-added canned white or red kidney beans |
| ½ | pound large shrimp, peeled and deveined |
| ½ | pound cod fillets, cut into ¾-inch pieces |
| 1 | cup fresh basil leaves, chopped |

**1.** Heat the oil in a large pot over medium heat. Add the celery and onion and cook for 6 minutes, stirring occasionally. Add the tomatoes, broth, zucchini, bell pepper, garlic, oregano, red pepper flakes, and beans. Bring to a simmer and cook for 10 minutes, or until the vegetables are just tender.

**2.** Stir in the shrimp and cod. Bring to a bare simmer, and cook for 5 minutes more or until the fish and shrimp are opaque. Stir in the basil right before serving.

MAKES 4 SERVINGS (2 CUPS PER SERVING).

**Per serving:** 251 calories, 28 g protein, 29 g carbohydrates, 4 g fat (1 g saturated), 8 g fiber, 451 mg sodium

# A Slice of Spaghetti
(pasta primavera pie)

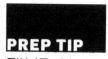

**PREP TIP**
## Fill 'Er Up

To add volume to drinkable yogurt without adding calories, pour it into a blender with some crushed ice and blend until smooth.

½    package (12.5 ounces) multigrain or whole wheat thin spaghetti

1    egg, plus 2 egg whites

⅓    cup finely chopped fresh parsley

⅛    teaspoon freshly ground black pepper

6    tablespoons grated Parmesan cheese

1    teaspoon olive oil

1    red bell pepper, chopped

½    pound asparagus, sliced ½ inch thick

2    cups frozen sugar snap peas, halved crosswise

3    large shallots, thinly sliced

1    clove garlic, chopped

2    tablespoons reduced-fat balsamic vinaigrette

¼    teaspoon salt

**1.** Cook the spaghetti according to the package directions and drain well. In a medium bowl, whisk together the egg, egg whites, parsley, ground pepper, and 3 tablespoons of the Parmesan. Add the pasta and toss together until evenly coated.

**2.** Heat the olive oil in a large nonstick skillet over medium heat. Add bell pepper, asparagus, peas, shallots, and garlic. Cook, stirring occasionally, for 8 minutes or until the vegetables are tender-crisp. Add the vinaigrette and salt to the skillet and toss to coat. Spoon into a medium bowl. Wipe out the skillet with a paper towel.

**3.** Coat the skillet with cooking spray and set it over medium heat. Add the spaghetti mixture and spread it evenly across the skillet. Cook for 3 minutes, or until golden brown. Loosen the edges and bottom of the mixture with a spatula.

**4.** Invert a large plate on top of the spaghetti mixture. Holding the plate in place, flip the spaghetti pie onto the plate. Coat the skillet with cooking spray and slide the pie back into the skillet, cooked side up. Cook for 3 minutes more.

**5.** Slide the pie onto a serving dish and cut it into 4 wedges. Spoon on the vegetables and top evenly with the remaining 3 tablespoons of Parmesan.

MAKES 4 SERVINGS (1 CUP OF VEGETABLES PER SERVING).

**Per serving:** 327 calories, 17 g protein, 54 g carbohydrates, 6 g fat (2 g saturated), 7 g fiber, 421 mg sodium

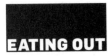

## Pick Up Sticks

When eating Chinese food, always use chopsticks. This automatically slows down the pace of your eating enough for your brain to signal your stomach that it's full before you overeat.

# No Worry Curry
(Thai chicken curry)

| | |
|---|---|
| 1 | pound boneless, skinless chicken breasts, halved lengthwise and sliced crosswise |
| 1 | large onion, halved and cut in ¾-inch pieces |
| 1 | large red bell pepper, cut into ¾-inch pieces |
| 1 | large green bell pepper, cut into ¾-inch pieces |
| 1 | cup diced pineapple |
| 1 | tablespoon julienned fresh ginger |
| 1½ | teaspoons curry powder |
| ¼ | teaspoon salt |
| ¼ | teaspoon crushed red pepper flakes |
| 1 | cup light coconut milk |
| 1½ | tablespoons honey |
| 1 | teaspoon cider vinegar |
| 2 | teaspoons cornstarch dissolved in ⅓ cup water |
| 2 | cups cooked brown rice |

**1.** Coat a large nonstick skillet with cooking spray and set it over medium-high heat. Add the chicken and stir-fry for 5 minutes or until browned. Transfer to a plate.

**2.** Coat the skillet with cooking spray. Add the onion and bell peppers. Cook, stirring, for 7 minutes or until tender-crisp. Stir in the pineapple, ginger, curry powder, salt, and red pepper flakes. Cook, stirring, for 1 minute.

**3.** Add the coconut milk, honey, vinegar, and chicken, along with any accumulated juices. Bring to a simmer and stir in the dissolved cornstarch mixture. Simmer for 2 minutes or until thickened. Serve with the brown rice.

MAKES 4 SERVINGS (1½ CUPS PER SERVING).

**Per serving:** 366 calories, 29 g protein, 45 g carbohydrates, 8 g fat (4 g saturated), 5 g fiber, 296 mg sodium

# Tex-Mex Pepper Steak Dinner
(chipotle glazed steak with black bean salad)

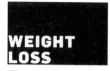

## Turn Your Back on the Buffet

Sit facing away from the all-you-can-eat buffet (and as far away as you can, too), and you'll be less tempted to go back for thirds.

| | |
|---|---|
| 1 | can (15 ounces) reduced-sodium black beans, rinsed and drained |
| 1 | cup frozen corn kernels, thawed |
| 2 | plum tomatoes, diced |
| 1 | avocado, diced |
| 1 | jalapeño pepper, seeded and finely chopped |
| 2 | tablespoons chopped cilantro |
| 2 | tablespoons fresh lime juice |
| $\frac{1}{2}$ | teaspoon salt |
| $1\frac{1}{2}$ | teaspoons salt-free chipotle seasoning blend |
| 1 | teaspoon packed brown sugar |
| 1 | pound sirloin steak, trimmed of visible fat |

**1.** Combine the beans, corn, tomatoes, avocado, jalapeño, cilantro, lime juice, and $\frac{1}{4}$ teaspoon of the salt in a medium bowl.

**2.** Preheat a grill or broiler. Mix the seasoning blend, brown sugar, and the remaining $\frac{1}{4}$ teaspoon of salt in a small bowl. Rub the spice mixture over both sides of the steak. Grill or broil the steak, 4 minutes per side for medium rare, turning once. Let rest 5 minutes. Thinly slice the steak and serve it with the black bean salad.

MAKES 4 SERVINGS.

**Per serving:** 373 calories, 31 g protein, 26 g carbohydrates, 17 g fat (4.5 g saturated), 9 g fiber, 418 mg sodium

## This Little Piggy Went to Athens
(pork gyros)

|   |   |
|---|---|
| 1 | teaspoon dried oregano |
| 2 | tablespoons safflower or olive oil |
| 2 | tablespoons red wine vinegar |
| 4 | cloves garlic, minced |
| 1 | pork tenderloin (1¼ pounds), trimmed |
| ¼ | teaspoon freshly ground black pepper |
| ½ | teaspoon salt |
| ⅓ | cup fat-free Greek yogurt |
| 2 | tablespoons chopped fresh dill |
| 4 | whole wheat pitas, halved and toasted, if desired |
| 2 | cups packed baby spinach leaves |
| 1 | tomato, cut into thin wedges |
|   | End of Summer Salad (see recipe on page 234) |

**1.** In a large, resealable plastic bag, combine the oregano with 1 tablespoon of the oil, 1 tablespoon of the vinegar, and all but ¼ teaspoon of the garlic. Add the pork, seal the bag, and turn the bag to coat the pork with the marinade. Let stand for at least 30 minutes in the refrigerator.

**2.** Preheat the oven to 425°F. Remove the pork from the marinade and discard the marinade. Season the pork with the pepper and ¼ teaspoon of the salt. Heat the remaining 1 tablespoon of oil in a large ovenproof skillet over medium-high heat. Add the pork and cook for 5 minutes, turning occasionally, until browned. Place the skillet in the oven and roast the pork for 15 to 20 minutes, turning once, until a thermometer inserted in the thickest portion registers 155°F and the juices run clear. Remove the pork to a cutting board and let rest for 5 minutes.

**3.** In a small bowl, combine the yogurt, dill, the remaining 1 tablespoon of vinegar, the remaining ¼ teaspoon of garlic, and the remaining ¼ teaspoon of salt.

**4.** Thinly slice the pork. Stuff the pita halves with the pork, spinach, and tomato wedges, and drizzle with the yogurt sauce. Serve with the watermelon-cucumber salad.

MAKES 4 SERVINGS.

**Per serving:** 362 calories, 37 g protein, 29 g carbohydrates, 11 g fat (1.5 g saturated), 4 g fiber, 635 mg sodium

# Roast Alaska
(roasted sockeye salmon with white bean compote)

| | |
|---|---|
| 1 | pound wild salmon fillet (in one piece) |
| 1 | pint grape tomatoes |
| 1 | tablespoon olive oil |
| ½ | teaspoon salt |
| ¼ | teaspoon freshly ground black pepper |
| 1 | can (15 ounces) reduced-sodium cannellini beans, rinsed and drained |
| ½ | cup roasted red and yellow peppers, chopped |
| ¼ | cup pitted kalamata olives, chopped |
| 1 | tablespoon lemon juice |
| ¼ | cup chopped fresh basil |
| 1 | teaspoon balsamic vinegar |

**1.** Preheat the oven to 425°F. Coat a rimmed baking sheet with cooking spray. Place the salmon on the prepared baking sheet. Arrange the tomatoes around the salmon. Drizzle the tomatoes with 1 teaspoon of the oil. Sprinkle the salmon and tomatoes with ¼ teaspoon of the salt and ⅛ teaspoon of the pepper. Roast for 12 to 15 minutes, or until the salmon is just opaque in the center and the tomatoes are soft.

**2.** While the salmon cooks, combine the beans, roasted peppers, olives, and lemon juice in a medium bowl.

**3.** Remove the tomatoes to a small bowl and stir in the basil, balsamic vinegar, the remaining 2 teaspoons of olive oil, the remaining ¼ teaspoon of salt, and the remaining ⅛ teaspoon of pepper. Cut the salmon into 4 pieces, discarding the skin. Serve over the bean compote with the roasted tomato mixture spooned over the top. Serve with sautéed escarole on page 234.

MAKES 4 SERVINGS.

**Per serving:** 342 calories, 29 g protein, 17 g carbohydrates, 11 g fat (2 g saturated), 4 g fiber, 716 mg sodium

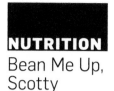

**NUTRITION**

## Bean Me Up, Scotty

A big pot of chili is the ultimate guy food, and it can be a big help when you're shedding your gut, too. It's loaded with beans (fiber), beef or turkey (protein), and hot peppers, which can encourage slower eating so you feel fuller, faster. Add the hottest sauce you've got. The spice will heat up your body and make you sweat, burning off a few extra calories. Best of all, chili is tough to screw up. The longer it cooks, the more stuff you throw in it, the better it tastes.

## Sautéed Escarole

1   tablespoon olive oil

2   cloves garlic, thinly sliced

1   bunch escarole, cut into 2-inch pieces

$\frac{1}{8}$   teaspoon salt

In a large nonstick skillet, heat the olive oil over medium heat. Add the sliced garlic and sauté for 30 seconds. Add the cut escarole and cook for 4 to 5 minutes, stirring frequently, until the escarole is wilted and tender. Stir in the salt and serve.

MAKES 4 SERVINGS.

**Per serving:** 54 calories, 2 g protein, 5 g carbohydrates, 4 g fat (0 g saturated), 4 g fiber, 101 mg sodium

## End of Summer Salad
(watermelon-cucumber salad)

2   cups diced seedless watermelon

$\frac{1}{2}$   cucumber, peeled, halved, and sliced

3   tablespoons crumbled feta

1   tablespoon red wine vinegar

In a medium bowl, combine the watermelon, cucumber, feta, and red wine vinegar. Toss gently to coat. Chill before serving.

MAKES 2 SERVINGS.

**Per serving:** 90 calories, 3 g protein, 13 g carbohydrates, 3 g fat (2 g saturated), 1 g fiber, 160 mg sodium

## Lazy Taters
(lightly mashed potatoes with cottage cheese)

| | |
|---|---|
| 1½ | pounds large red potatoes washed, but not peeled |
| 4 | tablespoons unsalted butter |
| ⅓ | cup skim milk |
| 8 | ounces cottage cheese |
| 1 | tablespoon red pepper flakes |
| | Salt and freshly ground black pepper |

**1.** Place the potatoes in a large pot and cover with water. Bring to a boil and cook until the potatoes are fork-tender, about 40 minutes.

**2.** Drain. Remove from the pot and cut into bite-size chunks.

**3.** Add the butter and milk to the pot and place over low heat to melt the butter. Dump in the potatoes, but don't mash them.

**4.** Add the cottage cheese, red pepper flakes, and salt and pepper to taste, and stir to combine. (The stirring will leave the potatoes more chunky than mashed.)

SERVES 6.

**Per serving:** 187 calories, 7 g protein, 21 g carbohydrates, 9 g fat (5.5 g saturated), 2 g fiber, 179 mg sodium

**WEIGHT LOSS**

The Sourpuss Diet

Eating grapefruit may help your body metabolize sugar and lower insulin levels, and a study in California showed that grapefruit helps obese people lose weight. People who ate half a grapefruit three times a day before meals lost nearly 4 pounds more than dieters who didn't eat grapefruit. The scientists speculate that grapefruit's acidity may slow the rate of digestion, keeping you feeling full longer and making you less likely to have seconds.

## Lose During Lunch

Make packing a lunch part of your morning routine and you'll dramatically reduce your calories consumed at work—and save some dough. Pack your lunch in a small, soft-sided cooler with a freezer pack to keep things cold, and be sure to include some snacks. Here's a sample menu:

■ An apple and two slices of cheese for a morning snack.

■ A 400- to 500-calorie portion of leftovers from the previous day's dinner.

■ A premixed protein shake or pint of milk and natural peanut butter rolled into a whole wheat tortilla for an afternoon snack.

## Chinatown
(rice bowls with shrimp and bok choy)

1   cup quick-cooking brown rice blend (such as brown rice, wild rice, Texmati white, and red rice)

3   tablespoons ponzu sauce

3   tablespoons rice wine vinegar

2   teaspoons grated, peeled, fresh ginger

2   teaspoons packed brown sugar

1   teaspoon sriracha sauce

4   teaspoons toasted sesame oil

1   head bok choy, thinly sliced

1   pound cooked shrimp

2   carrots, shredded

1   cucumber, peeled, halved lengthwise, seeded, and thinly sliced

$\frac{1}{3}$   cup fresh cilantro

**1.** Cook the rice according to the package directions, without added salt or fat.

**2.** In a small bowl, whisk the ponzu, vinegar, ginger, brown sugar, sriracha, and 3 teaspoons of the sesame oil.

**3.** In a large nonstick skillet, heat the remaining 1 teaspoon of sesame oil over medium heat. Add the bok choy and cook for 3 to 4 minutes or until wilted, stirring frequently.

**4.** Place the rice in the center of 4 bowls. Arrange the bok choy, shrimp, carrots, and cucumber around the rice. Drizzle with the dressing and sprinkle with the cilantro.

MAKES 4 SERVINGS.

**Per serving:** 319 calories, 30 g protein, 35 g carbohydrates, 7 g fat (1 g saturated), 4 g fiber, 698 mg sodium

# SWEET TREATS

We're lucky that baking desserts is so time-consuming, because otherwise we'd eat them too often. Here are some occasional treats.

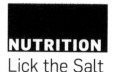

## NUTRITION
## Lick the Salt

Salt can cause you to eat unconsciously, which is why it's so easy to plow through a bag of chips. But you can beat your salt habit with just 2 weeks on a reduced-sodium diet.

### There's Newton to It
(apple-cherry spice bars)

|       |                                |
|-------|--------------------------------|
| 1     | cup unbleached all-purpose flour |
| $\frac{1}{2}$ | cup whole wheat flour      |
| 1     | teaspoon ground cinnamon       |
| 1     | teaspoon baking soda           |
| $\frac{1}{2}$ | teaspoon ground ginger     |
| $\frac{1}{4}$ | teaspoon salt              |
| $1\frac{1}{4}$ | cups unsweetened applesauce |
| $\frac{3}{4}$ | cup packed brown sugar     |
| 2     | tablespoons safflower oil      |
| 1     | cup dried tart cherries        |
| 1     | cup walnut pieces, chopped     |

**1.** Preheat the oven to 350°F. Line a 9 x 13-inch baking pan with foil, letting the foil extend over each edge of the pan by 2 inches. Coat the foil with cooking spray.

**2.** In a small bowl, whisk together the all-purpose flour, whole-wheat flour, cinnamon, baking soda, ginger, and salt.

**3.** In a large bowl, stir the applesauce, brown sugar, and oil until blended. Add the flour mixture to the applesauce mixture and stir just until combined. Stir in the cherries and walnuts.

**4.** Scrape the batter into the prepared pan and spread it evenly. Bake until a toothpick inserted in the center comes out clean, about 20 minutes. Place the pan on a rack and let it cool completely. Carefully lift the foil out of the pan and cut into 24 bars.

MAKES 24 SERVINGS.

**Per serving:** 114 calories, 2 g protein, 19 g carbohydrates, 4 g fat (0.5 g saturated), 2 g fiber, 79 mg sodium

## Cold, Dark, and Spicy
(blackberry-ginger frozen yogurt)

| | |
|---|---|
| 1 | pound blackberries |
| 1 | tablespoon grated fresh ginger |
| $\frac{1}{2}$ | cup fat-free vanilla yogurt |
| 2 | tablespoons honey |
| $\frac{1}{4}$ | teaspoon ground ginger |
| $\frac{1}{4}$ | teaspoon pure vanilla extract |

**1.** Combine the blackberries and fresh ginger in a blender or food processor. Blend or process until smooth.

**2.** Add the yogurt, honey, ground ginger, and vanilla, and mix to combine. Place in a covered bowl and refrigerate for about 40 minutes. When the mixture is cold, transfer it to an ice cream maker and follow the manufacturer's directions.

MAKES 4 SERVINGS (1 PINT).

**Per serving:** 109 calories, 3 g protein, 24 g carbohydrates, 1 g fat (0 g saturated), 6 g fiber, 22 mg sodium

## Puddin' It Off
(chocolate rice pudding)

| | |
|---|---|
| ½ | cup quick-cooking (instant) brown rice |
| 3¼ | cups 1% milk |
| ⅓ | cup sugar |
| 3 | tablespoons unsweetened cocoa |
| 3 | tablespoons cornstarch |
| | Pinch of salt |
| 2 | ounces bittersweet chocolate (70%), finely chopped |
| 1 | teaspoon vanilla extract |
| 1 | pound strawberries, hulled and sliced |

**1.** In a small saucepan, combine the rice and 1 cup of water. Bring to a boil, reduce the heat to low, and simmer, covered, for 10 minutes or until the rice is tender and the water has been absorbed. Add 1 cup of the milk and return to a simmer. Cook for 10 minutes, stirring frequently, until the rice is very tender and most of the milk is absorbed. Set aside.

**2.** In a medium saucepan, whisk the sugar, cocoa, cornstarch, and salt until well blended. Gradually whisk in the remaining 2¼ cups of milk until smooth. Cook over medium-low heat, stirring constantly with a heatproof rubber spatula, until the mixture thickens and comes to a simmer, about 10 minutes. Reduce the heat to low and cook for 2 minutes, stirring constantly. Add the rice and cook for 1 minute, stirring constantly. Remove from the heat. Add the chocolate and stir until it's melted. Stir in the vanilla and remove from the heat.

**3.** Pour the pudding into 8 dessert dishes. Place the dishes on a rimmed baking sheet and cover the surfaces directly with a sheet of plastic wrap. Refrigerate until cold, about 3 hours. Serve topped with the strawberries.

MAKES 8 SERVINGS.

**Per serving:** 170 calories, 5 g protein, 29 g carbohydrates, 4 g fat (3 g saturated), 3 g fiber, 85 mg sodium

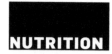

**NUTRITION**

## Root for the Bills

Have a bison burger (or an ostrich burger) while watching the game. These lean meats are packed with muscle-building nutrients and are tasty alternatives to ground beef.

## Tastes Like a Picnic
(watermelon sorbet)

4   cups cubed seedless watermelon

2   tablespoons lime juice

2   tablespoons stevia

Mint leaves

Pinch of sea salt (optional)

**1.** Combine the watermelon chunks, lime juice, and stevia in a blender and blend until smooth.

**2.** Pour the puree into a freezer container with a lid and freeze for 3 hours.

**3.** Spoon into small ice cream dishes and garnish with the mint leaves. Add a pinch of sea salt, if desired.

MAKES 4 SERVINGS (1 CUP EACH).

**Per serving:** 48 calories, 1 g protein, 13 g carbohydrates, 0 g fat (0 g saturated), 1 g fiber, 51 mg sodium

# Wookies
(chocolate-walnut wafer cookies)

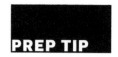

**PREP TIP**

Sweeten
the Deal

Add citrus fruits
or crushed frozen
berries to seltzer
water to add flavor.

- ¼ cup old-fashioned oats
- 1 cup unbleached all-purpose flour
- ½ cup unsweetened Dutch-process cocoa
- ¼ teaspoon baking soda
- ¼ teaspoon salt
- 4 tablespoons unsalted butter, softened
- ⅓ cup granulated sugar
- ⅓ cup packed brown sugar
- 1 large egg
- 1 teaspoon vanilla extract
- ½ cup chopped walnuts

**1.** Put the oats in a blender or food processor and blend or process until finely ground. Sift the flour, cocoa, baking soda, and salt into a medium bowl; stir in the oats.

**2.** In a large bowl, use an electric mixer on medium speed to beat the butter, granulated sugar, and brown sugar until creamy. Beat in the egg and vanilla until well blended. Reduce the mixer to low and beat in the flour mixture; stir in the walnuts.

**3.** Shape the dough into a 12-inch log and wrap it tightly in waxed paper. Refrigerate until firm. (A day or two is ideal, but wait at least 2 hours, if you're impatient.)

**4.** Preheat the oven to 350°F. Line a large baking sheet with parchment paper. Cut the log into scant ¼-inch slices and arrange them 1½ inches apart on the prepared baking sheet. Bake for 10 minutes, or until firm. With a spatula, transfer the cookies to a rack and let them cool. Repeat with the remaining dough, letting the baking sheet cool between batches.

MAKES ABOUT 5 DOZEN COOKIES.

**Per serving (2 cookies):** 70 calories, 1 g protein, 9 g carbohydrates, 3 g fat (1 g saturated), 1 g fiber, 33 mg sodium

# PART

# 4

## THE FAT BURNER'S
## BAG OF TRICKS

You've mastered the basics. Now it's time to turn up the heat.

In any workout or weight-loss program, you'll hit plateaus. They happen naturally when your body adapts to whatever program you're using. The secret to breaking any plateau is surprising your body, challenging your muscles, and forcing them to work in a different or more intense way. Professional athletes and their trainers learned this a long time ago and make it the foundation of their fitness philosophies.

That's also the fun of it: If you're constantly tweaking your workout and trying new exercises you've never done before, you'll never get bored. You'll look forward to your sweat sessions and you'll strive for even better results.

You have the talent; now you need the tools. In this section, you'll find a collection of inspiring tricks and tips from Belly Off! Club members, plus full-blown total-body workouts that are designed to challenge your muscles and optimize your body's metabolic burn. It's the next step in your physical transformation. You're going to look great. You'll feel even better. You can't stop now, because we mean it when we say the best is yet to come!

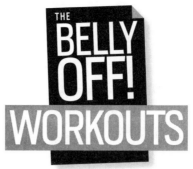

# Chapter 10

# THE KEEP-IT-SIMPLE
# DUMBBELL
# WORKOUT

## A Pair of Dumbbells and an Adjustable Bench Are All You Need to Drop Unwanted Fat and Add Eye-Catching Muscle

T he gleaming chrome machines of a gym may look high-tech and advanced, but they are actually quite limiting. Most allow you to perform what's called single-joint exercises, where your range of motion is limited to one plane. (Think leg extension, biceps curl, and bench press machines.) Because the machine is designed to lock you in to moving in

**GET JACKED!**

To make a dumbbell squat do double duty, perform a goblet squat with pulse:

Grasp a single dumbbell vertically by cupping one end of the weight with both hands. Hold the weight against your chest. Brace your abs and lower your body by pushing your hips back and bending your knees. Pause when your thighs are parallel to the floor and press the weight away from you until your arms are fully extended. Bring the weight back in to your chest and stand up. Do 8 to 10 reps.

—David Jack

only one direction at a time, only a small, targeted section of muscle actually receives the bulk of the resistance. That's better than nothing, but if you really want to build muscle mass and gain strength, training with free weights helps you develop your synergistic muscles—the wide range of little-known muscles that support the big-name muscles that you are trying to strengthen. Unlike resistance machines, free weights require you to balance the weight, which calls upon many more stabilizing muscles and makes the exercise that much more difficult, requiring greater exertion, which in turn burns more calories. And no free weight is better at that—or more versatile as a strength-building tool—than the simple dumbbell. Just learning how to bench press a pair of unwieldy dumbbells in a biomechanically efficient pattern takes skill, forces your muscles to adapt, and results in a deeper overall physical commitment.

The following workout was adapted from a dumbbell workout designed by Belly Off! trainer, fitness expert, and owner of TurbulenceTraining.com, Craig Ballantyne, CSCS, MS. All you need is a single set of dumbbells and an adjustable bench. The order in which you perform the exercises—along with the number of repetitions for each—allows the same pair of dumbbells to challenge each muscle equally. If you use a weight that allows you to do all reps without breaking form, then without a doubt, this is one of the simplest yet most effective workouts for chiseling a better body.

■ Perform three different dumbbell workouts each week, along with at least two 20-minute cardio workouts (walking, running, cycling, swimming), one interval-based, one steady-state aerobic.

■ Before each workout, complete two rounds of the warmup circuit described below. Advised but optional: the beginner Flex Series stretches on page 63.

■ Perform the exercises in the order on the chart on page 250. Alternate between the two exercises in each pair and complete all the sets in the first pair before moving to the next pair.

■ Cool down with one round of the active stretches on page 265.

■ Follow this workout program for at least 2 and ideally 4 weeks before moving to another workout.

## BODYWEIGHT WARMUP CIRCUIT

Complete the warmup circuit two times, resting for 30 seconds between circuits.

### Y-SQUAT
#### 10 REPS

Hold your hands overhead in a Y formation and place your feet greater than shoulder-width apart. Pushing your hips backward, squat until your thighs are at least parallel with the floor. Push back to the starting position.

### PUSHUP
#### 10 REPS

You know how to do this. (See page 72 if you need a refresher.)

## STICKUP
### 10 REPS

Stand with your back against a wall, feet 6 inches away from the wall. Stick your hands up overhead. Keeping your shoulders, elbows, and wrists in contact with the wall, slide your arms down the wall, bending at the elbows as you go, and tuck your elbows in at your sides. Return to the starting position.

## MOUNTAIN CLIMBER
### 10 REPS

Start in a pushup position. Keeping your head in line with your body, alternate bringing your right and left knees to your chest in a running motion as fast as you can. A right and left knee lift equals one rep.

## FORWARD LUNGE
### 10 REPS

From a standing position, take a large step forward with one leg. Bend your front knee until your front thigh is parallel to the floor and your back knee is near the floor; hold that position for 1 second. Return to the standing position and repeat with your other leg. That's 1 rep.

## WAITER'S BOW
### 10 REPS

Keep your knees slightly bent and your back arched naturally as you bend forward at the hips until your torso is parallel with the floor. Hold for a second. Return to the upright position.

## SPIDERMAN CLIMB
### 10 REPS

Start in a pushup position. Keeping your abs braced, pick your right foot up off the floor. Slowly bring your knee up and outside of your shoulder, and touch your foot to the ground. Slowly return your leg to the starting position. Repeat with your left leg. That's 1 rep.

# THE KEEP-IT-SIMPLE DUMBBELL WORKOUT

This 3-day-a-week total-body program contains three different dumbbell workouts: A, B, and C. Perform each workout once a week, resting at least a day between sessions. Within each workout, alternate sets between exercises of the same number (1A and 1B, for example) until you complete all sets in that pairing. (In other words, follow a set of the first exercise with a set of the second exercise.) Pay attention to how you rest during these circuits. For 1A and 1B, take a 1-minute rest between the two, as well as another minute after finishing 1B. For 2A and 2B, take *no* rest between them, but rest for 1 minute after you finish 2B. (This adds a nice metabolic circuit effect to the workout.)

Take care to use perfect form. Cheating by using momentum to help you lift the weight only compromises your progress.

Here's a sample workout schedule. You can start Workout A on any day of the week. Just be sure to leave at least a day in between workouts to rest and recover.

## Weeks 1 to 4

| MONDAY | TUESDAY | WEDNESDAY | THURSDAY | FRIDAY | SATURDAY | SUNDAY |
|---|---|---|---|---|---|---|
| Dumbbell Workout A | Rest / Walk | Dumbbell Workout B | Cardio Workout: 20-minute interval of your choice | Dumbbell Workout C | Cardio Workout: 30-minute steady-state aerobic | Rest / Walk |

# WEEKS 1 TO 4

## DUMBBELL WORKOUT A

### WARMUP

Bodyweight Circuit (2 rounds)

- Y Squat, 10 reps
- Pushup, 10 reps
- Stickup, 10 reps
- Mountain Climber, 10 reps
- Forward Lunge, 10 reps
- Waiter's Bow, 10 reps
- Spiderman Climb, 10 reps

Intermediate Flex Series (page 89) (1 round)

| STRENGTH EXERCISES | REPS | SETS |
|---|---|---|
| **1A DUMBBELL CHEST PRESS** | 8 | 3 |
| **1B DUMBBELL BENT-OVER ROW*** | 12 with each arm | 3 |
| **2A DUMBBELL SQUAT** | 8 | 2 |
| **2B DUMBBELL INCLINE PRESS**** | 15 | 2 |

*Rest 1 minute between A and B
**No rest between A and B

### COOLDOWN

Active Stretches (1 round)

- Walking Lunge, 10 reps
- Stickup, 10 reps
- Knee Hug, 10 reps each leg
- Corner Stretch, 3 10-second holds
- Walk in circles, 30 seconds
- Hamstring Stretch, 3 30-second holds each leg
- Groin Stretch, 3 30-second holds
- Cat/Cow Stretch, 5 reps

## WORKOUT A

# 1A DUMBBELL CHEST PRESS

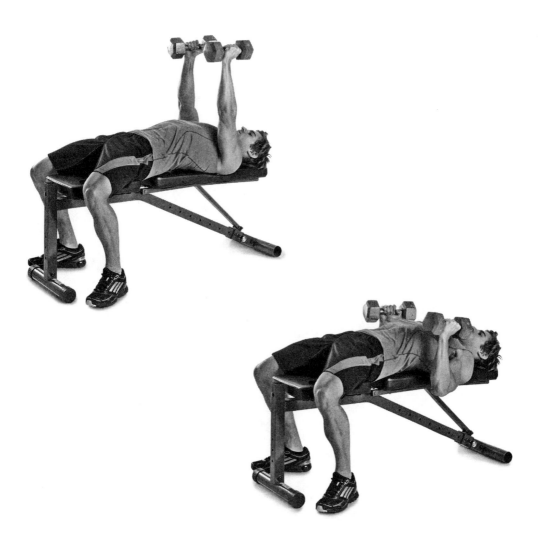

Lie on your back on a flat bench and hold a pair of dumbbells above your chest with your arms straight. Lower the dumbbells to the sides of your chest, pause, and then push them back to the starting position. Do 8 reps.

## WORKOUT A

# 1B DUMBBELL BENT-OVER ROW

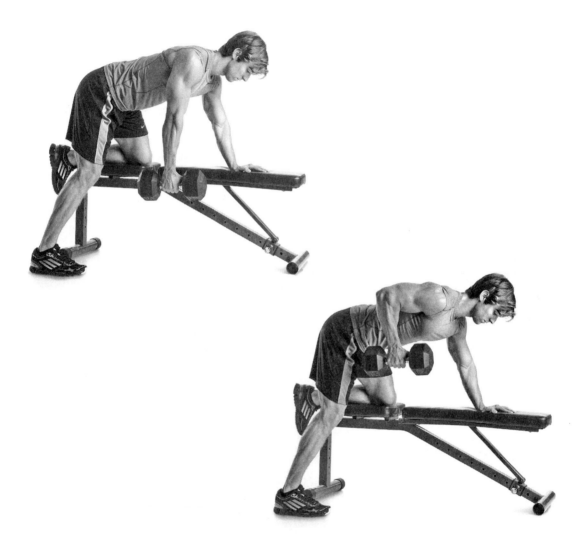

With a dumbbell in your right hand, place your left hand and left knee on a flat bench. Keep your back flat and let your right arm hang straight down, with your palm facing in. Pull your arm up to the side of your chest by bending your elbow. Pause, and return to the starting position. After 12 reps, switch sides, hold the weight in your left hand, and repeat the exercise.

## WORKOUT A

# 2A DUMBBELL SQUAT

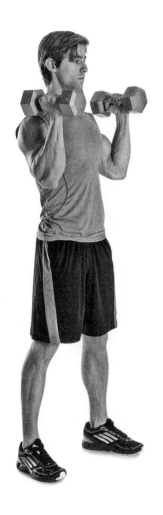

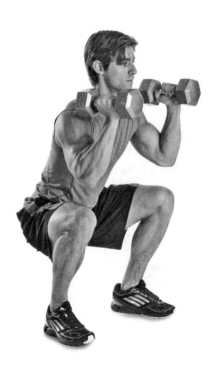

Holding a pair of dumbbells at your shoulders, stand with your feet just beyond shoulder-width apart. Push your hips back and squat down as far as possible, keeping your lower back naturally arched. Push back up to the starting position without rounding your back. Do 8 reps.

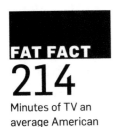

**FAT FACT**
# 214
Minutes of TV an
average American
watches on a typical
weekend.

**WORKOUT A**

# 2B DUMBBELL INCLINE PRESS

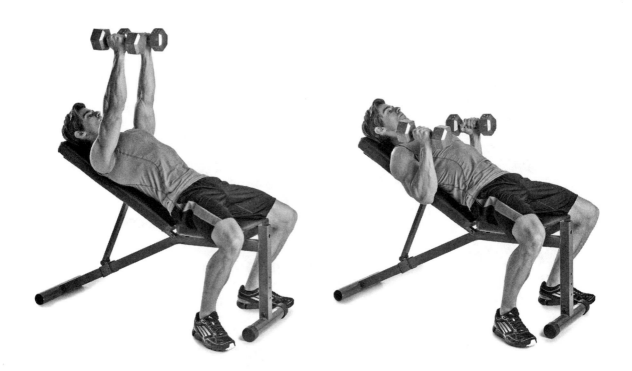

Lie on a bench with the backrest set at a 45-degree incline. Hold a pair
of dumbbells above your chest with palms facing in. Lower the weights
to chest level, then press them back to the starting position. Do 15 reps.

# WEEKS 1 TO 4

# DUMBBELL WORKOUT B

## WARMUP

Bodyweight Circuit (page 247), 10 reps
each exercise (2 rounds)

Intermediate Flex Series (page 89) (1 round)

| STRENGTH EXERCISES | REPS | SETS |
|---|---|---|
| **1A DUMBBELL SPLIT SQUAT** | 8 (each leg forward) | 3 |
| **1B DUMBBELL SINGLE-ARM STANDING SHOULDER PRESS*** | 12 (each arm) | 3 |
| **2A DUMBBELL ROMANIAN DEADLIFT** | 10 | 2 |
| **2B DUMBBELL SWING**** | 20 | 2 |

*Rest 1 minute between A and B
**No rest between A and B

## COOLDOWN

Active Stretches (page 265)

## WORKOUT B
# 1A DUMBBELL SPLIT SQUAT

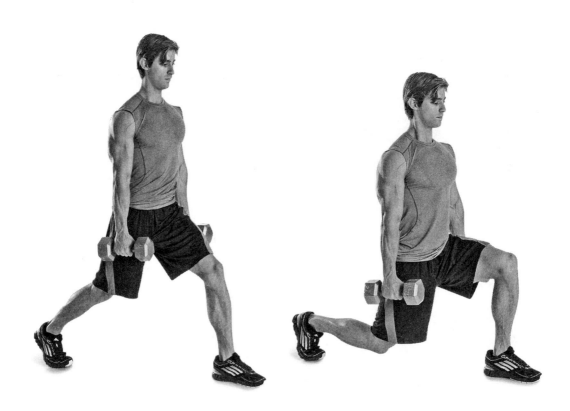

Hold a pair of dumbbells at your sides and stand with your left foot forward and your right foot back. Lower your body until your front knee is bent at 90 degrees and your rear knee nearly touches the floor. Return to the starting position. Do 8 reps, switch legs, and repeat. That's 1 set.

**WORKOUT B**

# 1B SINGLE-ARM STANDING SHOULDER PRESS

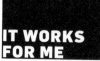

## IT WORKS FOR ME

"When my feet began hurting and I lost my breath walking up small hills, I thought, 'I'm going to die if I don't do something.' So on December 6, 2006, I grabbed a notebook and started a weight-loss journal. I wrote down my weight, what I ate that day, and the reasons I wanted to drop pounds: so I'd stop feeling like an embarrassment to my family, so I wouldn't need seat belt extenders on planes, so I'd prove everyone wrong. The journal helped me focus and think about losing weight every day."

—Tom Larsen
**Weight Before:**
353 pounds
**Weight After:**
200 pounds
The Belly Off! Club,
September 2009

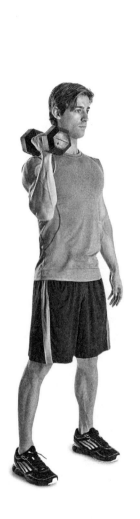

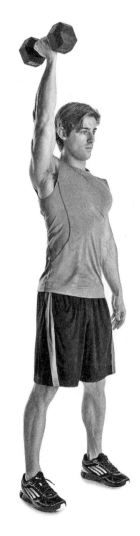

Stand holding a dumbbell at your shoulder, with your arm bent and palm facing inward. Press the dumbbell straight overhead, and then lower it to the starting position. Do 12 reps on one side, switch arms, and repeat. That's 1 set.

## WORKOUT B

# 2A DUMBBELL ROMANIAN DEADLIFT

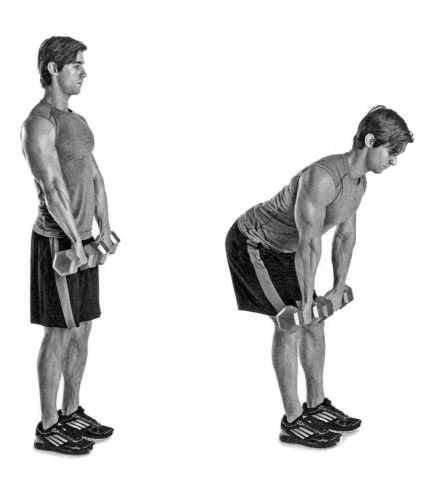

Hold a dumbbell in each hand in front of your thighs, palms facing your body. With your knees slightly bent and feet shoulder-width apart, bend at your hips and lower your torso until it's nearly parallel to the floor. Pause, and then rise to the starting position. Do 10 reps.

**WORKOUT B**

# 2B DUMBBELL SWING

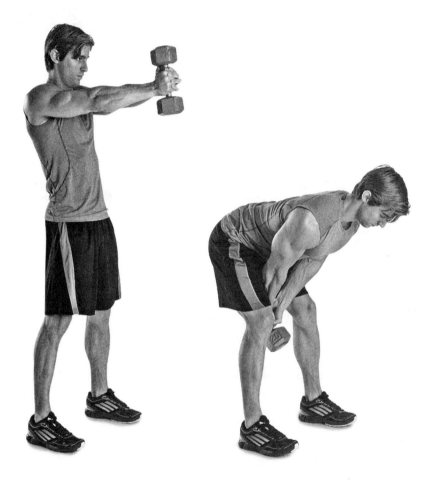

**FIT FACT**
Freestyle

The swimming stroke that provides the best workout for most people because it works the largest amount of muscle mass and can be executed for the longest amount of time and with the most intensity.

Stand with your feet shoulder-width apart and hold one dumbbell or kettlebell with both hands on the handle at arm's length in front of your chest. Bend at the waist and swing the weight down between your legs as if snapping a football, while keeping a flat back, your hips back, and your arms straight. Keeping your heels down and using your hips, glutes, and legs, "pop" your hips forward while swinging the weight up to eye height. Focus on controlling the weight. Brace your core and hold your breath on the down swing and release a tense breath swinging the weight up. That's 1 rep. Do 20.

# WEEKS 1 TO 4

# DUMBBELL WORKOUT C

## WARMUP

Bodyweight Circuit (page 247), 10 reps
each exercise (2 rounds)

Intermediate Flex Series (page 89) (1 round)

| STRENGTH EXERCISES | REPS | SETS |
|---|---|---|
| 1A DUMBBELL STEPUP | 8 | 3 |
| 1B DUMBBELL CHEST-SUPPORTED INCLINE ROW* | 12 | 3 |
| 2A DUMBBELL CURL | 10 | 2 |
| 2B DUMBBELL LYING TRICEPS EXTENSION** | 12 | 2 |

*Rest 1 minute between A and B
**No rest between A and B

## COOLDOWN

Active Stretches (page 265)

## WORKOUT C

# 1A DUMBBELL STEPUP

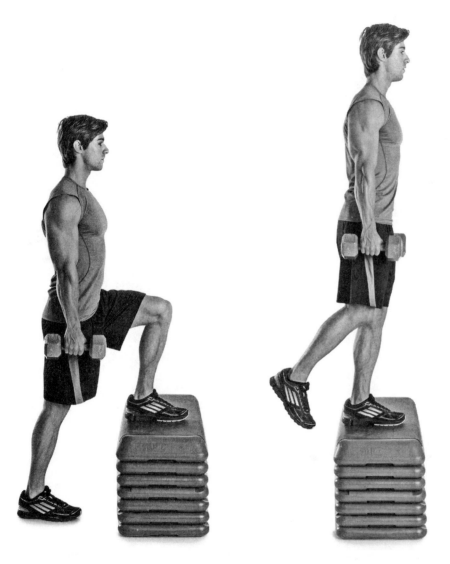

With a dumbbell in each hand, stand facing a bench. Place one foot flat on
the bench. Press through your foot to lift your body up to the standing position
without letting your opposite foot touch the bench. Lower your body slowly
and repeat. Complete 8 reps, switch legs, and repeat. That's 1 set.

## WORKOUT C

# 1B CHEST-SUPPORTED INCLINE ROW

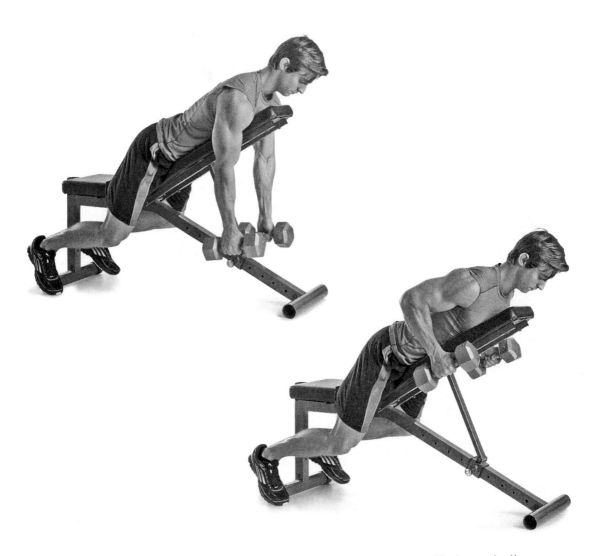

Grab a pair of dumbbells and lie chest-down on a 45-degree incline bench. Let your arms hang straight down, palms facing each other. Row the dumbbells to the sides of your chest by bending your elbows and squeezing your shoulder blades together. Pause and lower the weights. Do 12 reps.

## WORKOUT C

# 2A DUMBBELL CURL

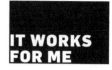
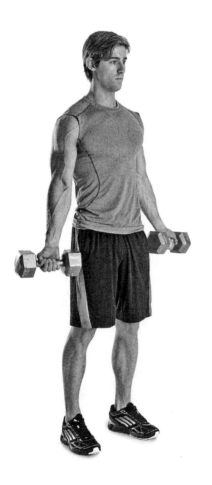
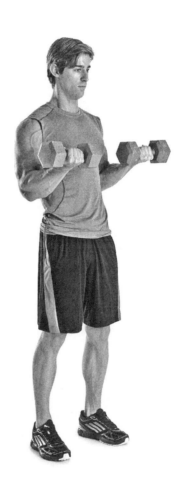

Grab a pair of dumbbells and hold them at arm's length next to your thighs, palms facing forward. Curl the dumbbells toward your chest as far as you can without moving your upper arms. Pause, and slowly lower the weights to the starting position. Do 10 reps.

**FITNESS**
Lift
Backward

When you become
bored with a
workout, inject some
variety (and confuse
your muscles) by
reversing the order
in which you do your
exercises.

**WORKOUT C**

# 2B LYING DUMBBELL TRICEPS EXTENSION

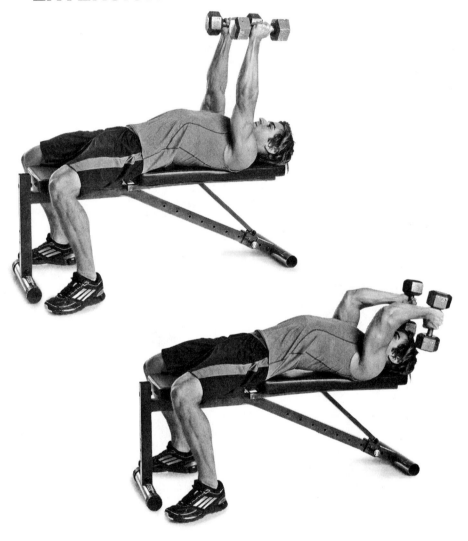

Lie on a flat bench holding a pair of dumbbells above your chest, palms facing in. Keeping your upper arms still, bend your elbows and slowly move the weights toward your ears. Straighten your arms back to the starting position. Do 12 reps.

## COOLDOWN

These active stretches will help you recover from the workout and keep you flexible and injury-free. Do them after your workout in the following order:

- Forward Lunge, 10 reps (see page 248)
- Stickup, 10 reps (see page 248)
- Knee Hug, 10 reps with each leg
- Corner Stretch, 3 reps, each held for 10 seconds
- Walk in large circles while shaking out your arms and legs for 30 seconds
- Hamstring stretch, 3 reps, holding each stretch for 30 seconds
- Groin stretch
- Cat/Cow Stretch (see page 35)

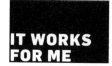

**IT WORKS FOR ME**

"Do the exercises you dread. The ones that get you groaning the most pay off best. Just sticking with the easy stuff won't give you results. Also, make your fitness public. Signing up for a 5-K or a weekly ball game with the guys will give you constant motivation to push yourself in the gym."

—Josh Bone
**Weight Before:** 310 pounds
**Weight After:** 180 pounds
The Belly Off! Club, March 2008

## SUCCESS STORY

## Cut Out the Beer

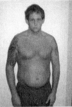

**Weight Before**
### 270

**Weight After**
### 170

# JOE BINKLEY
NORWALK, OH
THE BELLY OFF! CLUB, DECEMBER 2010

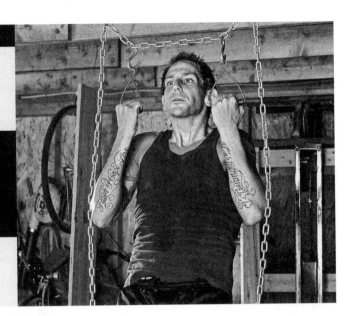

### THE WAKE-UP CALL
Most guys pig out in high school. Me? I practically starved myself. I'd grown up a heavy kid, and that was the only slimming strategy I knew. When I turned 21 and became a bartender, I swung to the other extreme: Tons of junk food and alcohol made my body balloon. I guzzled energy drinks to stay alert at work, which helped for a while. My sales were so good that my boss promoted me to the bar's busiest section, but I couldn't keep up. Sales slipped. I was demoted. My body felt broken.

I spent years trying random diets, but my weight only yo-yoed.

Finally I realized that I couldn't just cut out things like late-night Taco Bell runs—I had to cut out the thing that caused me to make those runs in the first place: alcohol.

### HOW I CHANGED
As I researched healthy eating, I realized that I needed a mix of carbohydrates, protein, and healthy fat—and that nutritious food could fuel me far better than energy drinks could. So I switched to six small, well-balanced meals a day. Now a meal is a chicken breast with vegetables and a snack is a banana with peanut butter. And most important, I cut out booze entirely.

Once I decided to

lose weight, I vowed to run a local 4-mile race. I started training slowly—alternately running and walking three or four times a week until I was able to run half an hour straight. Six months later, I finished the race in just over 36 minutes. After that I became active in local races and logged 11 to 18 miles a week.

I also started lifting weights and now I'm hooked on powerlifting and bodybuilding. I've intentionally bulked up to 193 pounds. This is very different from my weight loss. Now I'm eating 6 to 10 meals a day, roughly 3,600 calories, to fuel my extremely intense workouts. My mind

now is so driven to make sure I eat correctly and train daily that I have to fight it when I need a day off from the gym.

### THE REWARD
I never went back to drinking. I'm not a teetotaler, it just isn't for me and has serious implications for an individual's health. Today, I am a nutrition consultant for GNC and I recently graduated from Bible college with a focus on children's ministry. I realized how deeply ingrained fitness can become in your life. Powerlifting, bodybuilding—they're a crucial part of my life, like my faith. And I feel fortunate to have found that out.

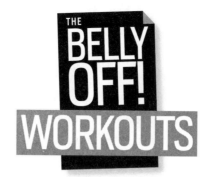

# Chapter 11

# THE FAT TORCH

## Fell Off the Fitness Wagon? This Density Training Workout Will Help You Rebound in 30 Days!

Sometimes life intervenes and you drop out of an exercise routine. Happens all the time. It's really easy to do: You get ultrabusy at work. You move to a new house or change jobs. Somebody leaves an infant on your doorstep, and suddenly catching up on sleep takes priority over the Belly Off! Advanced workout.

The belly comes back. The muscles get soft. Willpower and determination hibernate for the winter, and you reach for the Christmas cookies.

A 4-week metabolism reboot can quickly put you back on track after even months off the fitness wagon. Thirty days is just the right amount of time to commit to finding your path back to fitness. Not too long, not too short. You haven't been away from exercise for so long that you need to start from scratch, but you also need something substantial that you can commit to, something with a reward at the end. It's times like these when our Fat Torch workout, a program of 16 workouts (4 each week for 4 weeks) is the perfect way to reverse weeks of body neglect. It's a beautiful thing because it's a short workout that's easy and works fast. It employs density training, a technique that allows you to do more work in less time. You'll sweat enough to raise sea levels and you'll bring your muscles back up to form quickly, so you can return to the Belly Off! Advanced workout. It's also an awesome workout for those who want to shape up fast for the beach or a special occasion. Four weeks is all it takes.

**WORKOUT 411**

■ Perform two different workouts—A and B—4 days a week for 4 weeks. Each workout includes six exercises, which are paired. You will do as many sets of each pair as possible in 10 minutes.

■ Do workouts A and B back to back, take a rest day off, then repeat A and B.

■ Restart the same schedule the following week.

■ Begin each workout with a warmup of your choice, plus the Intermediate Flex Series.

■ End each workout with a 3-minute walk, plus the Intermediate Flex Series.

■ Use your choice of Belly Off! Walking Interval Program schedules (page 23) as your daily cardio plan.

# Weeks 1 to 4

| MONDAY | TUESDAY | WEDNESDAY | THURSDAY | FRIDAY | SATURDAY | SUNDAY |
|---|---|---|---|---|---|---|
| Strength Workout A | Strength Workout B | Rest | Strength Workout A | Strength Workout B | Rest | 60-minute Endurance Walk |

# Strength Workout A

For each exercise pairing (1A and 1B, for example), alternate back and forth after each set. Five repetitions equal 1 set. Use a weight that you can lift 10 times with good form, but remember to only do 5 reps. (Don't worry: It'll be quite challenging.) Complete as many sets of the two exercises as possible in 10 minutes. Rest for 2 to 3 minutes and then move on to the next pair of exercises.

## WEEKS 1 TO 4
## STRENGTH WORKOUT A
### WARMUP
Your Choice + Intermediate Flex Series (page 89)

| STRENGTH EXERCISES | REPS | SETS |
|---|---|---|
| 1A GOBLET SQUAT | 5 | As many as possible of 1A and 1B in 10 minutes |
| 1B CHINUP | 5 | |
| 2A DUMBBELL PUSH PRESS | 5 | As many as possible (each arm) of 2A and 2B in 10 minutes. |
| 2B DUMBBELL BENT-OVER ROW | 5 | |
| 3A ALTERNATING DUMBBELL BENCH PRESS | 5 | As many as possible of 3A and 3B in 10 minutes |
| 3B JUMP SQUAT | 5 | |

## COOLDOWN
Walk for 3 minutes + Intermediate Flex Series (page 89)

# 1A GOBLET SQUAT

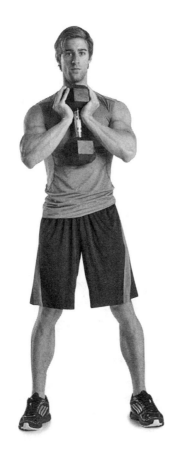

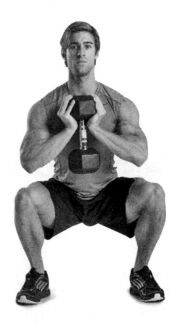

Hold a dumbbell vertically next to your chest, with both hands cupping the dumbbell head. Brace your abs and lower your body as far as you can by pushing your hips back and bending your knees. Pause, and then push through your heels to return to the starting position. Do 5 reps.

# 1B CHINUP

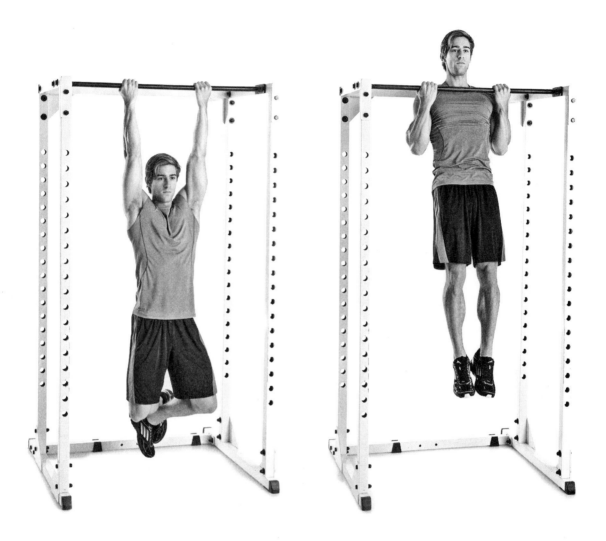

Grab a chinup bar with a shoulder-width, underhand grip, and hang at arm's length. Pull your chest up to the bar. Once the top of your chest touches the bar, pause, and then slowly lower your body back to the starting position. Do 5 reps.

# 2A DUMBBELL PUSH PRESS

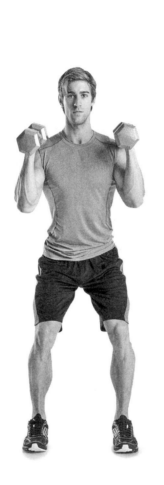
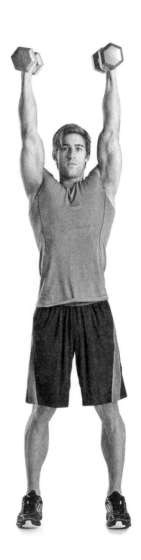

Stand holding a pair of dumbbells next to your shoulders with your elbows bent and your palms facing each other. Dip by bending your knees slightly, and then push up with your legs as you press the dumbbells over your head. Lower the dumbbells back to the starting position. Do 5 reps.

# 2B DUMBBELL BENT-OVER ROW

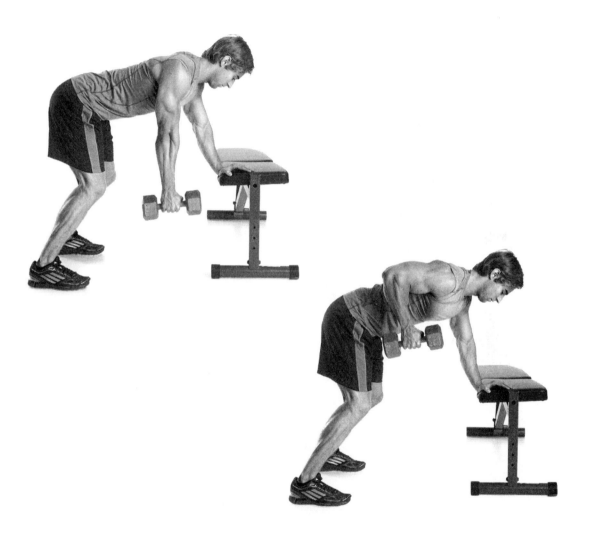

With a dumbbell in your right hand, place your left hand on a flat bench. Keep your back flat and let your right arm hang straight down, with your palm facing in. Pull your arm up to the side of your chest by bending your elbow. Pause, and return to the starting position. Do 5 reps, then repeat the exercise with the dumbbell in your left hand.

# 3A ALTERNATING DUMBBELL BENCH PRESS

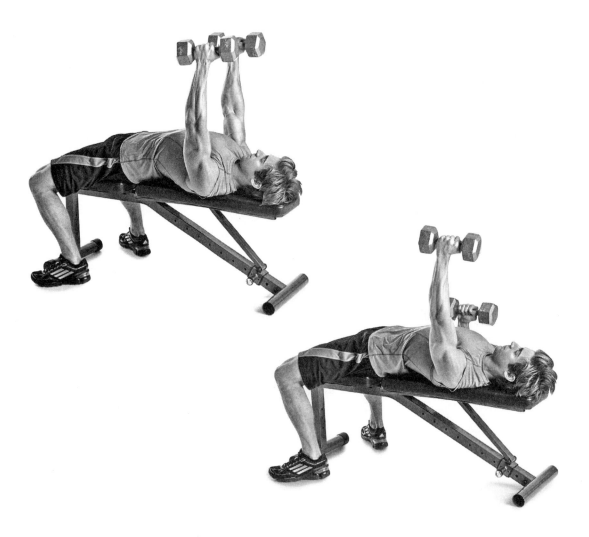

Grab a pair of dumbbells and lie on your back on a flat bench, holding the dumbbells over your chest with your arms extended straight up. (You can use a neutral grip, as shown, or position your palms facing your feet.) Lower one dumbbell to the side of your chest, and then press the weight back to the starting position. Switch arms and repeat. That's 1 rep. Do 5.

# 3B JUMP SQUAT

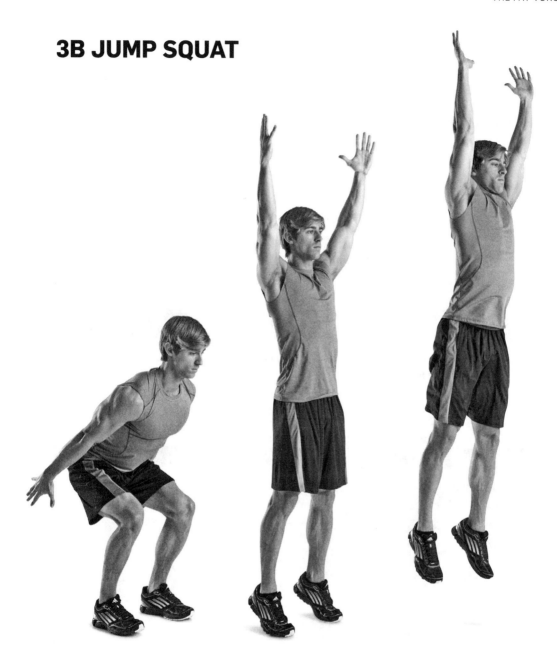

Stand tall with your feet shoulder-width apart, and then lower your body as far as you can by pushing your hips and arms back. Pause, and jump as high as you can. When you land, immediately squat down and jump again, without pausing. Do 5 reps.

# Strength Workout B

Perform these 6 exercises as a circuit, doing 10 repetitions of each exercise and resting for 30 seconds before moving to the next one, one after another until all of the exercises have been completed. That's 1 round. Complete a total of 3 rounds. Try to increase the weight you use each week.

## WEEKS 1 TO 4

## STRENGTH WORKOUT B

### WARMUP
Your Choice
Intermediate Flex Series (page 89)

| STRENGTH EXERCISES | REPS | SETS | ROUNDS |
|---|---|---|---|
| CIRCUIT | | | 3 |
| DUMBBELL HANG PULL | 10 | 1 | |
| DUMBBELL PUSHUP AND ROW | 10 | 1 | |
| REVERSE LUNGE AND SWING | 10 | 1 | |
| HIGH-KNEE RUN | 10 | 1 | |
| DUMBBELL SWING | 10 | 1 | |
| CROSS-BODY MOUNTAIN CLIMBER | 10 | 1 | |

### COOLDOWN
Walk for 3 minutes
Intermediate Flex Series (page 89)

# DUMBBELL HANG PULL

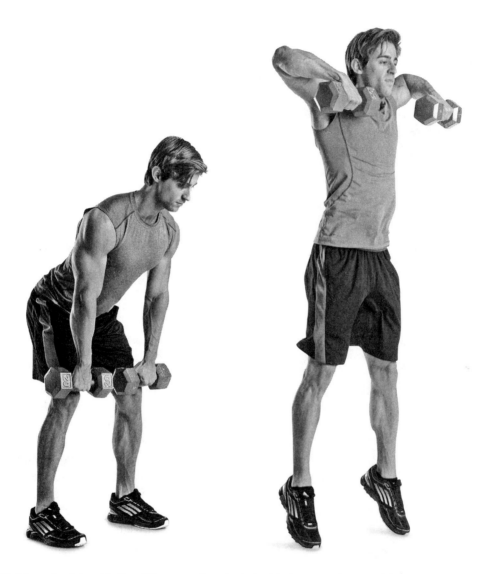

Hold a pair of dumbbells with an overhand grip just below your knees with your hips pushed back and your knees slightly bent. Pull both dumbbells to shoulder height by thrusting your hips forward and standing up on your toes. (Avoid leaving the ground.) Return to the starting position, pause, and repeat. Do 10 reps.

# DUMBBELL PUSHUP AND ROW

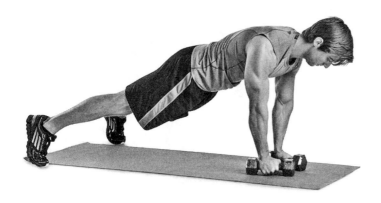

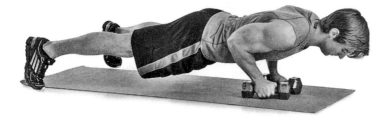

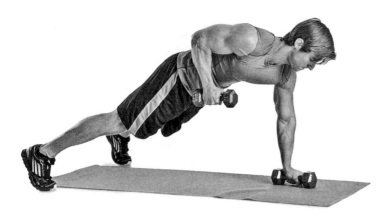

Place a pair of dumbbells on the floor, shoulder-width apart. (We suggest using hexagonal dumbbells so they won't roll.) Grab the handles and get into a pushup position but spread your feet for balance. Do a pushup, then row the dumbbell in your right hand to the side of your chest. Lower your right arm to the starting position and row with the dumbbell in your left hand. That's 1 rep. Do 10.

# REVERSE LUNGE AND SWING

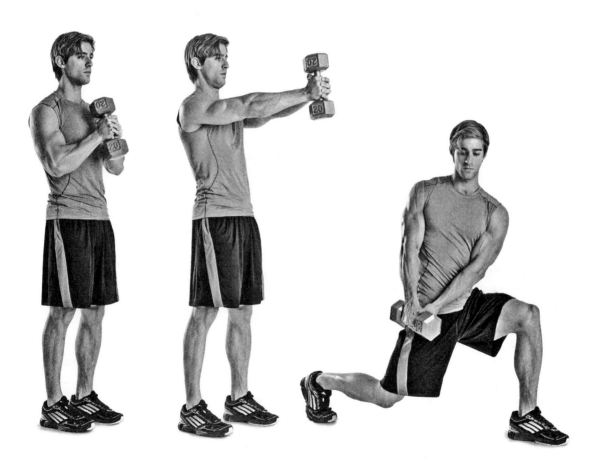

Hold a dumbbell with both hands in front of your chest and then press the weight straight out in front of you. Lunge back with your right leg as you rotate to your right and swing the dumbbell to your right hip. Then push back to a standing position as you swing the dumbbell back to eye level. Next, do the reverse lunge with your left leg and swing the weight to your left hip. That's 1 rep. Continue alternating sides for 10 reps.

# HIGH-KNEE RUN

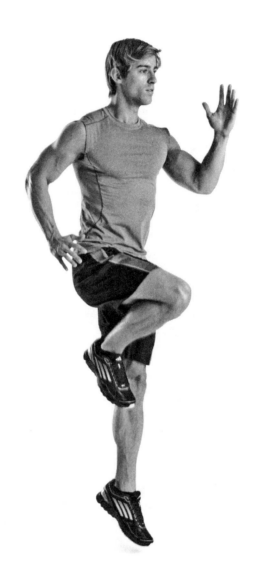

Stand tall and run in place as fast as you can. Drive through the balls of your feet and try to bring your heels up under your backside so that your knees go high toward your chest. Keep your hands relaxed, elbows bent, and shoulders down, and swing your arms back and forth. A high-knee on your left and right legs equals 1 rep. Do 10.

# DUMBBELL SWING

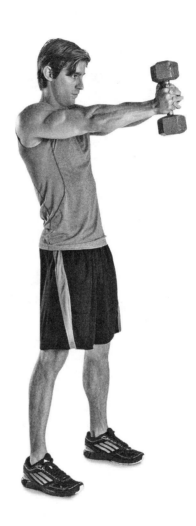

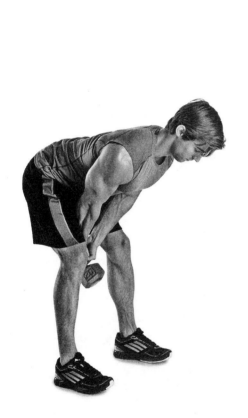

Stand with your feet shoulder-width apart and hold one dumbbell or kettlebell with both hands on the handle at arm's length in front of your chest. Bend at the waist and swing the weight down between your legs as if snapping a football, while keeping a flat back, your hips back, and your arms straight. Keeping your heels down and using your hips, glutes, and legs, "pop" your hips forward while swinging the weight up to eye height. Focus on controlling the weight. Brace your core and hold your breath on the down swing and release a tense breath swinging the weight up. That's 1 rep. Do 10.

# CROSS-BODY MOUNTAIN CLIMBER

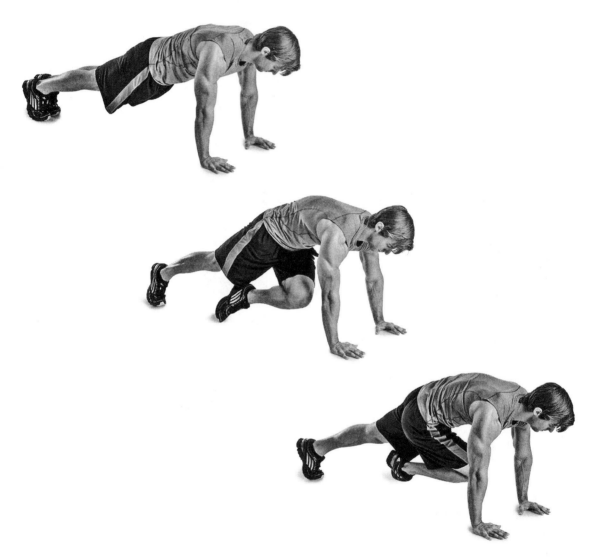

Get into a pushup position with your arms straight. Lift your left foot off the floor and bring your left knee under your body and toward your right elbow. Return to the starting position and bring your right knee toward your left elbow. That's 1 rep. Repeat, alternating legs quickly. Keep your hips level and don't pause during the exercise. Do 10 reps.

# The Tool Shed

## BEST FITNESS GEAR TO STOCK IN YOUR HOME GYM

Convenience has a way of inspiring results. So does free membership and not having to wipe someone else's sweat off a bench. If you've been doing the Belly Off! workouts, you know that they are designed for home use and they don't require a ton of weights and other equipment. But having a few pieces of the right gear at your disposal can certainly expand your exercise options and accelerate your results. Here are some of the best tools for building muscle and torching flab from the comfort of anywhere—your home, your office, a hotel room—even the gym, if you're so inclined.

# RESISTANCE BAND

How can a giant rubber band help you build muscle? Simple: Unlike a barbell or dumbbell, a resistance band provides constant tension throughout a lifting movement, increasing the intensity of the exercise and the challenge to your muscles. It's not the best way to add tons of bulk (free weights are still tops for that), but it's a fast, portable way to gain real-world strength.

If you buy one pair, go with the Purple Large Bands from Resistance Band Training Systems; they provide 50 to 75 pounds of resistance ($45). If it's variety you're after, buy the Intermediate Band Package, which has four pairs ranging in resistance from 15 up to 120 pounds, for $100 more. resistancebandtraining.com

**BEST EXERCISE**

# BAND OVERHEAD REVERSE LUNGE

Stand with your feet shoulder-width apart, loop the band under your left foot, and press the ends of the band overhead until your arms are straight. That's the starting position. Keep the band pressed overhead as you lunge backward with your right leg until your front knee is bent 90 degrees and your back knee is an inch or two off the floor. Return to the starting position. That's 1 rep. Do 3 sets of 12 reps, switching legs halfway through each set.

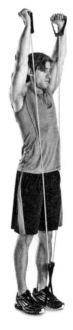
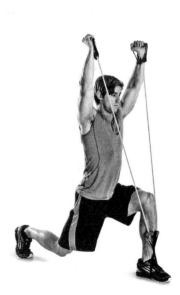

# MEDICINE BALL

Today's medicine balls swap leather for easier-to-grab vinyl, but there's a reason the basic design hasn't changed for decades: It's one of the most dynamic strength builders you can own. It's also one of the few designed to leave your hands. Hurling it against a wall or the ground engages nearly every muscle in your body—especially those in your core.

The Dynamax 8-pound Accelerator 1 Ball is designed to absorb impact, so it won't rocket back up into your face when you do medicine ball slams (see below). It's also made from 70 percent recycled materials. If you want room to grow, pick up 12- and 16-pound balls, as well. $85, medicineballs.com

**BEST EXERCISE**

## MEDICINE BALL SLAM

Grab a medicine ball in both hands and hold it above your head with your feet shoulder-width apart and your arms slightly bent. Now reach back as far as you can and slam the ball to the ground in front of your feet. Grab the ball on the rebound if it bounces. Otherwise, pick it up and repeat the movement. Do 3 sets of 12 reps. Want to make it harder? Stand on one leg and try to maintain balance and good form as you do the exercise.

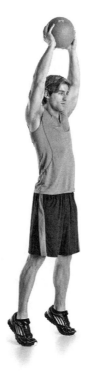
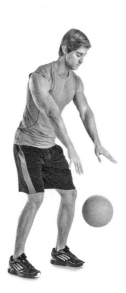

# KETTLEBELL

This Russian import looks like a cannonball with a handle, but that ungainly design is exactly why it's so effective. Unlike a dumbbell, a kettlebell's center of gravity shifts during an exercise, increasing the challenge and building coordination. And because it's intended for total-body moves, it adds a cardio element to what is already an intense strength workout.

We like the 16-kilogram First Place Kettlebell (about 35 pounds). There are more expensive brands with vinyl covers and nonskid bases, but this basic cast iron bell is all you need to build serious muscle. Want two? Add a 24-kilogram bell (about 53 pounds) to your order. $60 and $80, performbetter.com

**BEST EXERCISE**

## SINGLE-ARM KETTLEBELL SWING

Grab a kettlebell using an overhand grip and hold it with one hand, arm extended, at waist height. Set your feet slightly more than shoulder-width apart. Swing the bell between your legs as you bend at the waist and bend your knees. Keeping your arm straight, thrust your hips forward, straighten your knees, and swing the bell up to chest level as you rise to a standing position. That's 1 rep. Do 3 sets of 20 to 30 reps, switching hands halfway through each set.

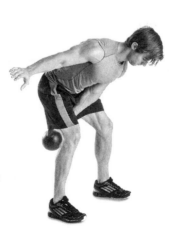
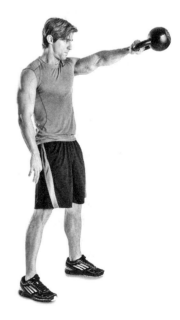

# SWISS BALL

Think of a Swiss ball as the opposite of solid ground—a soft, unstable surface that challenges your core and helps you improve your balance and coordination. It's also an excellent substitute for a bench in exercises like the chest press and the pullover, as long as your goal is to build coordination and stability rather than raw power and strength. Used alone, it's just about the best tool you can own for sculpting a six-pack.

Fitball Sport Stability Ball is available in a range of sizes, depending on your height, but the 65-centimeter model (26 inches) is a good fit for most men. Its latex-free vinyl construction can also support up to 600 pounds. $29, performbetter.com

## BEST EXERCISE

## SWISS BALL JACKKNIFE

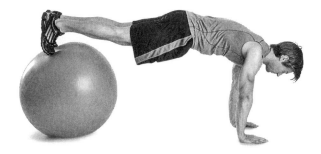

Get into a pushup position with your arms straight underneath your shoulders and your shins on a Swiss ball. Your body should form a straight line from your ankles to your head. This is the starting position. Without changing your lower-back posture, roll the ball toward your chest by pulling it forward with your feet. Pause, then lower your hips and roll it back to the starting position. That's 1 rep. Do 3 sets of 8 to 10 reps.

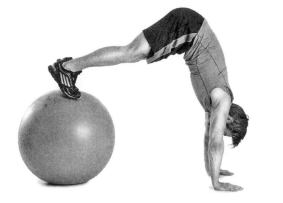

# SAFETY SCREEN:
# REVEAL YOUR WEAK SPOTS

## This self-test will identify everything from muscle imbalances to potential injury risks.

Assess your own readiness for exercise by answering the following questions.

**1.** Do you have any nagging injuries or chronic pains, especially in a bone or joint?

**2.** Have you had a recent and/or major injury to a muscle, bone, or joint?

**3.** Do you feel pain when you exercise, play sports, or are active?

If you answered yes to any of these questions, then you are in pain. We don't train in pain. We strongly encourage you to see a practitioner to get cleared for the workouts in this book. You can choose to see a corrective exercise specialist, like a physical therapist, or an integrated wellness professional, or your family doctor.

Next, perform these basic tests to identify any pain or areas of concern in your ankles, knees, hips, back, shoulders, and neck. Be honest. Ignoring pain will only lead to more pain. A doctor or good physical therapist can clean these issues up quickly.

- **Squat screen:** Perform a bodyweight squat. Do you feel pain in your hips, back, or knees?

- **Lying hamstring screen:** Lie on your back in a doorway and place one leg on the wall next to the door. Keep both legs straight and your down leg in contact with the ground, toe pointing up toward the ceiling. Continue to work your way further into the doorway, forcing your raised leg to go higher and create more of a stretch in your hamstring while keeping your body, head, shoulders, and hips on the ground. Take note of how far your leg can stretch. Perform the same test on the other side. Were you able to stretch as far? Did they feel different? If one leg is slightly tighter than the other, spend some time each day stretching that side with this test.

- **Ankle screen:** Stand with your head, shoulders, hips, and toes facing a wall, and place your hands against it. Put your left foot forward, placing your toes about 3 inches from the wall. Keeping your left heel down, gently drive your knee toward the wall, keeping it over your shoelaces. If you can keep your heel down and your knee touches the wall, back up a bit until your knee can just barely touch the wall. Mark that spot. Using your other foot, perform the same test. If either mark is much closer to the wall, or you feel pain, you'll need to work on improving mobility in your tighter ankle. Lack of mobility here will affect your entire body, from the ground up. Try the ankle circles described on page 64.

- **Back screen:** Lie facedown on the floor. Keeping your hips on the ground and lightly squeezing your glutes, press your torso away from the floor with your hands, as if you're entering Cobra Pose. Do you feel pain in the joints of your low back? Now get on all fours and sit your backside on your heels, with your arms extended out in front of you on the floor. Do you feel pain in this position? This is known as extension and flexion of the spine. If you experience joint pain in either position, you should discuss it with your doctor or physical therapist before starting the strength portion of this program.

- **Shoulder screen:** Extend both arms out to your sides, making loose fists. Without jerking, try to take one arm up and over your shoulder and the other arm down and under the opposite shoulder, and touch your fists in the middle of your back. Try the other side. Were your fists much further apart on one side (they will often be a bit further apart when your dominant hand is under the other), or did you feel any pain in your shoulders? If the answer to either question is yes, you will need to work on your shoulder flexibility.

- **Neck screen:** Look up, look down (putting your chin to your chest), look left, look right, try to touch your right ear to your right shoulder, your left ear to your left shoulder. Do you lock up in any of these motions? Do you feel pain?

How you fare on these tests will give you a good idea of whether you need to have a doctor or physical therapist intervene before embarking on the Belly Off! workouts.

During exercise, if you feel any pain, shortness of breath, or dizziness, stop exercising immediately and see a doctor. If you feel pain in a joint or bone within the first days after starting a new routine, stop or change the activity that seems to be causing the pain.

Know your body and listen to what it tells you, and you'll achieve the greatest success at changing your body safely.

# INDEX

Underscored page references indicate sidebars and tables. **Boldface** references indicate photographs.

INDEX **295**